health
is here

health
is here

ELENA SHEA, MD

Library of Congress Control Number: 2013901306
ISBN: Hardcover   978-1-4797-8382-3
                   Softcover   978-1-4797-8381-6
                   eBook   978-1-4797-8383-0

This book is for education and inspiration only and is not a substitute
for seeking medical care and adequate medical attention.

To order additional copies of this book, contact:
Xlibris LLC
1-888-795-4274
www.Xlibris.com
Orders@Xlibris.com
598589

Contents

INTRODUCTION

It is becoming increasingly important for us to know how to improve our health with our own efforts. As health care costs escalate, we cannot rely solely on Western medicine approaches and pharmaceuticals for our well being. Not only for our own quality of life, we must make active effort to improve the abilities and quality of life for our children starting in the home as teachers and guides for our children as well as setting an example for others. Today, more than ever, our environment is polluted with obstacles of every kind in the healthy development of our precious children. We must be aware of these exposures and depleted foods to recognize them. Therefore in this book, I am sharing what I have learned in an effort to strengthen the weak vessels many of us live in.

It is increasingly difficult to make good food choices, which are necessary for adequate growth and development. Obesity is rising at an alarming rate, and although we recognize inactivity as one of the causes, little effect is made on this rising health risk.

Attention deficits and depressions are also rising at alarming rates, and there is little association to these with diet in much contemporary medicine, which has been trained to use pharmaceuticals, an omnipresent industry.

As I stated, health begins in the home. Having a clean an environment as possible (not clean in the light of the various housecleaning chemicals) as fresh pure air, minimal dust and smoke, and fresh, pure water are all essential for healthy development. As parents, we can benefit our children greatly by taking the time to teach them lifestyle practices that will bring life and not death. This should not be an effort to have a perfect body but to maximize the vitality of the one you were given.

We all have personal weaknesses we must accept, boundaries unique to each of us. It is important to recognize these as well, not every person tolerates the same diet or can develop the same intellect, but each person also has unique gifts as well. I have also found that our weaknesses may become our greatest strengths when we respond to them appropriately. Sometimes our weaknesses shift us in a direction we might otherwise not go unless prompted in this way, a direction that ultimately serves God in a more profound way. Weaknesses are wonderful in that we rely on God's strength to overcome them, a power that we really cannot fully comprehend. They humble us in a way that nothing else can. They give us a sense of compassion and empathy that others cannot understand. They profoundly and permanently develop our spirit to maturity. Of course, this all occurs when we respond to these weaknesses effectively. We should not see these weaknesses as failures of our health efforts but realize the general weakness inherent in our current gene pool. This is not to say we should just give up and let these weaknesses destroy us, but we should continue to search for ways we can overcome our obstacles, seeking God's will all the while.

Teachers and schools also play a pivotal role in the development of our children, and sometimes, parents rely too much on this role of the schools, failing to do their part in raising their children. Especially younger children, they identify strongly with caring, friendly teachers who like them and want to see them do well. My children have been blessed with such schools. Most teachers I would believe go into this profession because of their inherent love for children and desire to make a difference in lives. Our teachers can augment the teachings of home but only if they too are aware of the problems within our diet.

The school lunches should be overhauled. With so much information on nutrition available to us, our school lunches are archaic. I understand a big problem is that children simply will not eat healthy foods a lot of the time, but we should make a serious effort to improve the quality of the foods children are exposed to at school. Is the lettuce devoid of any green? Are there any unprocessed foods at all available? What is the quality of the oil used in the pizza, chicken nuggets, or enchiladas? What is the quality of the meat? Has the beef been cooked sufficiently? What about the oils in the chips, rancid? Partially hydrogenated? What is the truth about milk? Are our children getting sodas at school? What about candy? We must be educated and attempt to educate our schools. Better nutrition means better behavior and learning ability. Many of our children are attempting to learn and be competitive with severe nutritional handicaps limiting their mental and physical development. Again, not all children will develop the same physical prowess or intellect, but we should strive to maximize what they do have. This is a continuous process that needs consideration and adjustments unique to each of our children. Some basics can be applied to all alike.

Be sure our children get plenty of fresh air and sunshine. Make purified water available to the children on a regular basis, send them with a water bottle and/or purify the water at schools. Encourage our children to drink this water, which tastes better than the chemical-laden water from the city. Simplify the beverages, add lemon or lime for flavor. Avoid rancid oils at all costs and teach our children to recognize them. Use minimally processed products and vegetables more regularly and limit the availability especially of red meats. Start these children out young and possibly limit their risks of chronic disease later, as well as improve their function and vitality now. Minimize candies and sweets, which deplete our children's nervous system and other tissues of valuable minerals and nutrients. Supply these nutrients and minerals regularly, especially when our children get the candy or sweets.

There are many considerations when raising children in our culture today. We are in a fast-moving, transient environment unlike in the past. Our foods and exposures are increasingly harmful to our wellbeing, and we should be especially aware of the changing forces upon our youth. We can have healthy children by being aware of inherent constitutional weaknesses and promoting nutritional habits; we can go a long way in improved vitality and physical and emotional function. Learning ability is improved and behavior responds favorably when lifestyle measures are addressed, especially when from an earlier age. As we become adults, it is harder to back track and restore vitality and function. It becomes more difficult to change habits as time goes by. It certainly is not hopeless though, children tend to respond more quickly to therapy and nutrition. There is always room for improvement. Also, we should not live in unnecessary guilt for things we are unaware of. It certainly is not my intention to arouse guilt but to educate.

The gastrointestinal tract is the cornerstone for providing adequate nourishment. Approaching our nutritional needs begins with understanding digestion, absorption, and assimilation. Indeed gastrointestinal illnesses are extremely common, affecting younger and younger individuals. Promoting health begins at the digestive tract. Bowel issues are costly and damage quality of life. There is so much hope for people willing to take more responsibility in their health and learn about natural approaches used for centuries and even millennia.

Our problem with bowel disease is increasing at an alarming rate, being related to our stressful, malnourished, and toxic world of today. Genetics play a role, and our generations have deteriorated in their vigor. The gastrointestinal tract is perhaps the most directly affected organ system with the changes in our food supply.

Symptoms of bowel disease can be vague or severe or anywhere in-between. Fatigue, nausea, bloating, burning, belching, pain, irritability, aches and pains, and obvious malnutrition can all manifest. Weakness in our digestion can eventually lead to problems in other organ systems, as well as weaken our general vitality and productivity. Efficient digestion is paramount in maintaining health.

We are tempted to say the diseases of today are related to our longer life span and may choose to deny the existence of toxins, pollutants, depleted soils and foods, pathogens, and other insults including those that have occurred earlier along the generational line. What I am suggesting is the weaknesses and imbalances not addressed in this generation may further adversely affect our descendants.

It can be from fear or inconvenience that we choose to ignore the reality of pollutants, toxins, and depleted food sources. This is not self preserving to carry these attitudes and not take personal responsibility for our health. For most of us, our personal choices in what we eat and are exposed to have great impact on our overall health. There are those who have very strong constitutions than are able to "get away" with poor habits, but generally, they too pay the price in their health and well being.

Lack of knowledge and cultural prejudice by patients as well as physicians can play a significant role in the confusion regarding the causes of disease and the role of herbal medicines in maintaining and securing health. The different approaches to healing should be combined more as illnesses have become even more complicated and diverse. Many of the same illnesses occurred historically when we approached the situation with foods and plants more readily. Knowledge of herbal success was obliterated by the pharmaceutical frenzy in which we are in the midst of today. Pharmaceutical medications certainly have improved health situations for many individuals. But now, we all want a simple pill to resolve our problems. We are increasingly finding that a simple pill doesn't work though. By not taking initiative to find the cause or multiple causes and addressing these, our health will continue to deteriorate no matter how many pills or "Band-Aids" we place. Combining knowledgeable approaches have a better chance at restoring and improving health.

There are many who want to make a difference, especially for the children and the sick. You cannot underestimate the role diet and medicinal plants play in healthcare. You may eventually not even need pharmaceutical medications at all with your wellness. The pharmaceutical industry may be threatened by these unpatentable medicines that might be grown in our own backyards. They should not worry so much though, there will always be a need for pharmaceutical medications; many will continue to choose these to avoid having to take some responsibility, and some disease states will need pharmaceuticals for at least a long period of time if not permanently even with proper diet and plant use. Illnesses often take a long time to present themselves, and thus, it takes a long time for them to reverse. There is no magic bullet.

Vitality

Vitality is a major factor in our quality of life. Vitality includes not only our energy but also our inherent resistance to stress and disease, a result of balanced functions in the body.

Many factors play into and affect our vitality and may be in our control to at least some extent. These include diet, environment, water supply, crowding, rapid transit, and expansion. All these and other influences affect how we feel, how effective we are. Unfortunately, there is a loss to disease.

Western medicine unfortunately has moved away from building vitality toward the symptom management of disease. As responsible persons, we should strive to improve not only our own lives but also, and even especially, the lives of others through our relationships. We can do our part to heal.

By covering symptoms only, often with pharmaceutical medications, we may ultimately limit and resist natural processes of the physical body. This potentially prevents any attempt at self-correction by the body. As our defense mechanisms are curtailed, our vitality is trimmed away. For example, according to Chinese medicine principles with its long history of evolution, antibiotics are cooling medicines thus potentially weakening an already depleted individual, although there is certainly a need and demand for them. For example antibiotics and corticosteroids are obvious causes of yeast overgrowth, a cause of disease yet to be fully understood, that should be approached with probiotics and even medications.

By addressing underlying issues and possible causes, we can attempt to reverse the illness process. Examples include eating nutritious, well-tolerated, and healing foods and plants, as close to the bottom of the food supply preferably. These foods such as soybeans, beans, fruits, vegetables, herbal teas can do much to maintain an alkaline body status. Alkaline blood is well maintained by a complex buffering system; a total body pH or acidity is all inclusive of every cell of the body. Body acidity, or pH less than 7, suggests a higher risk in in the development cancer and of autoimmune symptoms while total body alkalinity, the pH greater than 7, relatively is neutralizing, which supports health. White flour/white sugar products, for example, are acidifying while soy is definitely alkalinizing. Strong meats such as red meats tend to be acidifying because of breakdown products, but if chewed thoroughly, salivation can be quite alkalinizing alone. Have your lemon water before your meal.

This may take time; it has taken a long time to get into the situation we currently find ourselves in. Of course, prevention is ideal; but often, we do not become aware of the issues until symptoms are demanding our attention. Because of this, we frequently must address lifestyle and dietary habits aggressively and seriously to restore vitality, especially in the chronically ill. Severely ill patients may be too weak to undergo too many changes at once, and these cases it is wise to start slow but not to give up. Help the delicate individuals, juice the vegetables for them, or provide fresh juice to the very ill. People tolerate different juices differently, but generally, carrot, grape, vegetable and berry juices all have their value. Considerations such as diabetes need to be allowed for.

About Me

I have suffered from some form of autoimmune syndrome. Too long to really know. To let you understand my position and outlook, my mother was a very ill woman. Still is today, although she is still around but very limited in her health. Her twin is equally ill, as is a cousin of mine from that twin. My brother died of heart disease with a multitude of autoimmune complaints at the age of thirty-seven. I believe with all my heart that you cannot truly understand a person's diseased condition without direct firsthand or at least second-hand experience. I have been severely deathly ill. I am here to share the insights, wins, and losses of this ordeal.

If I can save one child from progressive disease, one individual from multiple surgeries or organ damage, one person's life, at least improve the quality of a person's life, or even allow for one person to taper down their prednisone and other toxic pharmaceuticals, I have done a big thing. I am a healer; this is my passion. To understand and have this purpose can be overwhelming but very satisfying.

After medical school, I completed my internship in 1993. From there I practiced family medicine with my mentor, the late Dr. Max Morales, a most loving, gentle, and giving physician. He knew of my mother who had autoimmune disease, of my own health that still was relatively good despite the exhaustion, and gently took me under his wing. After a year there, I moved on to urgent care, a love of mine. I learned much. My boss there also was a kind, gentle, highly respected person; he wanted to supply the best medicine he could in these clinics, and they prospered well until the billing department failed. Fortunately, many of the urgent cares are still operating well under the leadership of the individual doctors, and a big need in this Texas community is being met.

I learned a lot in the busy clinics I worked in. I became quite expert at picking out lung pathologies, heart pathologies, wound care, eyes, fractures, infections of various sorts, and more. I was in the trenches, as doctors would say. I gained a lot of insight into a variety of health issues and their effects on the sufferers.

After roughly eight years in urgent care with an excellent reputation, I decided I needed to stay home with my young children. My health was an issue, and the children needed a stable and calm environment as well; they are distinctly delicate as probably are all children. I could not provide that being distracted with work and my limiting health. All four of my children have GI symptoms, especially the three younger girls. If I do not figure this thing out, they are destined to a lifetime of the misunderstandings and misinformation. I stayed home, read, rested, played mommy, house, and learned about healing. This had been one of the most intense times of growth. After six years of staying at home and studying, caring for my children, I returned to complete a family medicine residency. I became board certified in family medicine in 2010 while I opened my own private practice. This experience continues to reinforce and educate me on healing. I have witnessed without any doubt the benefits to many patients. Their quality of life is undeniably improved. They heal faster, feel stronger, and understand themselves more fully. I want to share this knowledge with as many as will listen, as I see whole families improve in their own health.

There are many individuals who do not understand the alternative philosophy of medicine or wish too. It is unfortunate, but there will always be people not ready for new or actually old healing techniques. Prior to my generation of doctors, there was a paternalistic approach: the doctor knew everything and patients wholly relied on his advice (usually men). Now patients question doctors more; and unfortunately, doctors do not know everything, especially in regards to alternative, complementary, or substitutive care, whatever you choose to call it. There is absolutely so much knowledge available; it is a lot to sift through the pharmaceutical literature alone, much less looking into the history of authoritative books on healing.

In addition, doctors must stay in strict "standards of care" established, probably originally for the patient's protection, but now maintained for the insurance's protection, as well as the pharmaceutical industry's protection. This limits the physician's creativity and growth. That is one reason why we now have so many "health-care providers." Unfortunately, no patient fits in a book, and each needs individual approaches to their problems.

Medicine will always be an art as much as a science, and cookbook medicine eliminates the art. The art of healing does not belong to just physicians but to anyone willing to learn these historical uses of herbal medicines. Ideally, physicians of traditional training themselves will continue to see the benefit of appropriate herbs and reactions to herbs by proper usage. The proper uses of plants coupled with lifestyle modifications have possibilities and potential that is undeniable.

Chapter 1

Basic Digestion

Our digestive system is especially critical for maintaining health. This system is responsible for providing adequate nourishment as well as removing waste products. When this system is functioning, optimum health is supported, when the system is under stress and inefficient, various illnesses and symptoms can occur.

The digestive system in its entirety includes from top to bottom: the mouth, the pharynx, the esophagus, the stomach, the small intestines, the liver, the pancreas, the spleen, the large intestine and the rectum. Each individual organ has direct function in digestion.

The salivary glands are extremely important for alkalinizing the food and starting the breakdown of sugars in particular. We underestimate the importance of these glands, as we do many glands. To maintain healthy salivary flow, you should drink plenty of pure water between meals, leaving fewer liquids for mealtimes in an effort not to dilute the salivary secretions. Chew well also, this stimulates salivation and begins digestion. An easy remedy is lemon in water a half hour or so before your meal; let the water pass out of your stomach, which should not take too long in most cases if there is no food to slow it down. The lemon is particularly beneficial not only in stimulating saliva but also liver function, further supporting effective digestion. Bitters also early in a meal such as salad greens are quite helpful in stimulating digestion.

The stomach has two valves called sphincters. One is at the top of the stomach and one is at the bottom. The valve at the top of the stomach is called the lower esophageal sphincter (LES, at the bottom of the esophagus.) This valve is responsible for closing the top of the stomach. The breathing muscle, the diaphragm, which helps the valve to close efficiently, supports the LES valve. Sometimes the diaphragm is only loosely surrounding the LES that may cause the sphincter to not close as effectively. For some individuals, this causes heartburn, or acid leaking into the esophagus, especially when the foods are causing excessive acid. The other valve is the pyloric valve.

After the food is swallowed, it enters the stomach; the openings close, and acid and other digestive enzymes bathe the food, now termed a bolus, to especially break apart protein and large molecules. This supports concepts of food combining, discussed in a later chapter. This acid is necessary; we take way too many acid blockers, many that are extremely potent. Acid is also necessary to protect against pathogenic invaders, so without adequate acid, we invite these organisms. Acid, if not allowed to breakdown protein, leads to fermentation production in the large intestine where many bacteria await any undigested food. Diarrhea is a manifestation of mal-digestion and suggestive of pathogenic overgrowth. To go a little deeper, these bacterial and other secreted toxins from fermentation get absorbed into the blood and tissues, leading to conditions of toxicity of various systemic symptoms. Therefore, let us not assume we do not need acid because it is hurting us; let us get down to why the acid is bothering us. You should not rapidly stop any acid blocker though if you have been using them in any type of regular basis, you need to change habits and then remove the medicine, as you do not have the need for it anymore. Food combining and food allergens most certainly play a role in excessive acid problems, as well as poor food choices themselves (alcohol in excess.)

The second stomach valve, or sphincter, is at the end of the stomach, the pyloric sphincter. In a small proportion of babies, they are born with a condition in which the pyloric valve is very tight, causing excessive symptoms of burping and vomiting, as the stomach cannot empty properly. In these infants, they must undergo dilation procedures to open up the pyloric region more effectively; if this is not done, the babies may suffer growth delay as well as significant pain and irritability. Fortunately in mild cases, the baby may grow out of the problem. In some individuals, the pyloric valve may become irritated, swollen, and inflamed. This in turn causes poor stomach emptying as well, leading to the same symptoms of belching and vomiting as well as pain.

After the stomach, we reach the small intestine where bile from the liver greets juices from the pancreas to help further digest foods, now in particular, sugars, starches, and further protein breakdown as well as fats. In problems where the stomach is emptying too rapidly, as in poor food combining habits, the pyloric valve has opened too soon. This causes symptoms of indigestion as poor breakdown occurs to the damaged sugars. If the pyloric valve opens too slowly from poor food combining, putrefaction also occurs as the stomach acid does not appropriately break down meats.

The small intestine is quite important; it has multiple glands and absorptive capabilities and is quite long as a result. Food is now termed "chyme" because of the enzymes and bile that have been added for digestion. Yeast and other pathogens may overgrow here and in the large intestine further down the digestive tract, leading to leaky bowel discussed later. The small intestine ends at the cecum, a small pouch that opens into the large intestine with a valve near the appendix. This is one of those misunderstood glands; we may assume the appendix is a relic from past needs, but its immune function is still very much present as identified by microscope as well as in understanding the nature of glands. The appendix is full of immune cells and glandular structures.

When the chyme enters the colon (the large intestine) the main function here is the absorption of specific nutrients such as minerals, vitamins, as well as absorption of water, and storage and elimination of waste materials. Waste products are not only from breakdown of food particles and sloughing of intestinal cells, a normal turnover of approximately two weeks, but also from secretions from the liver as well as cells lining the colon. After storage in the large intestine, the water is reabsorbed along with bile salts, and the remainder is sent through the sigmoid portion of the colon to the rectum for elimination. The rectal sphincter is responsible for the voluntary ability to evacuate. It is important to evacuate when you feel the need, not to wait hours for a more convenient time. Holding bowels for prolonged periods may contribute to constipation in our later years. Get in the habit of having regular bowel movements of three a day if possible, and eat foods to encourage this pattern. If your problem is already there, there are many healing plants available.

Foods that encourage bowel movements:

1. Prune juice
2. Fruits
3. Bitter foods such as salad greens
4. Pure water between meals
5. Magnesium rich foods such as blueberries

Organs necessary for proper digestive process other than the direct digestive tract:

1. Liver, gallbladder
2. Pancreas
3. Spleen

Liver

The liver is so extremely important to health, not only in digestive processes but also almost more importantly in detoxification processes covered more thoroughly in chapter 6. The liver not only processes the absorbed food materials, the liver creates bile that is necessary for fat absorption. Bile is necessary to "emulsify" or break apart the fat molecules for better absorption. Bile also stimulates bowel motility as well as allows for waste removal. Bile carries away fat-dissolved contaminants into the large intestine to be later excreted.

The liver also manufactures many proteins and other substances necessary for digestion and absorption. The liver is responsible for the manufacture of so many vital nutrients for survival. Fortunately, the liver has an amazing capacity to heal itself, especially with support. This is so important in this age because of all the toxicities, infections, and alcohol issues that bombard the liver.

The liver receives its blood supply from two sources. The portal circulation brings in blood from the intestines that include many nutrients for use as well as wastes for modification. The hepatic circulation comes from the arterial tree, bringing oxygen to the tissues and removing carbon dioxide, the waste of "breathing" metabolism.

Herbs especially useful for liver support include milk thistle, which promotes cellular regeneration as well as protection to the cell structures within the liver. Dandelion is also a favorite of mine, so readily available. It is important though to collect the plant from safe environments, ones in which harmful chemicals such as pesticides and weed killers have not been applied for years. The entire plant is beneficial not only to the liver but the kidneys as well. The leaves are loaded in potassium, and the plant not only supports liver detoxification but also kidney function, allowing for diuresis safely on the level of the pharmaceutical furoseamide (brand name Lasix), a very powerful diuretic. The fantastic thing about dandelion, other than how cheap and available it is and the multiple benefits it provides, is its potassium of organic nature which naturally provides protection against potassium deficiency, so common with pharmaceutical diuretics. Barberry is another fantastic liver plant, stimulating detoxification function and bile flow. The docks, in particular yellow dock, also have remarkable liver stimulating support. Bitter herbs also include horehound and gentian that greatly stimulate liver activity and bile flow. Castor oil compresses are beneficial over the liver being quite stimulating and supporting for liver function.

If you are dealing with gallstones, remember gravel root and collinsonia, two well-recognized stone dissolvers. Gravel root can be invaluable with stones.

Also, considering the liver, the Chinese clock places the liver's best function to be roughly at 11 p.m. Having the foods available for assimilation is important for efficient liver function. On the other hand, eating late heavy meals detracts energy from the liver to the other portions of the digestive tract, impairing liver function.

Pancreas

The pancreas has two very important distinct functions to provide energy. Two distinct gland types accomplish this; the exocrine glands secrete digestive enzymes into the intestines while the endocrine glands on the "islets of Langerhaans" secrete hormones, mostly insulin, directly into the blood to manage blood sugar availability for cellular use. When digestion is impaired or blood sugar is erratic, pancreatic support is helpful.

Here you think of glandular herbs, mullein flowers and leaves come to mind. Other known herbs to support pancreatic function include cedar berries. Cedar berries (*Juniperus monosperma*) have been successful in lowering blood sugar historically for diabetic patients. Licorice root also is supportive for pancreatic function; this herb should be used in modest doses over a longer period of time than the doses required to control the inflammation. Licorice root in larger doses may raise blood sugar. For pancreatic support, licorice root is invaluable.

Good nutrition contributes to pancreatic enzyme production. Super foods loaded in minerals such as kelp, spirulina, and blackstrap molasses all especially support pancreatic function.

With the pancreas, as well as the rest of the digestive system, it is good to have rest periods between meals. This allows for regeneration of enzymes just as rest for us allows our body to heal. Constant snacking is not recommended.

Spleen

The spleen is generally unrecognized as important for the digestive processes. I have included this organ because of my understanding of Chinese and other Eastern medicine placing tremendous importance on this organ for its absorption and storage capacities, which are very poorly understood in Western medicine. Here we believe we really do not need a spleen as we should. The spleen in Chinese medicine is the yin to the stomach, storing the energy obtained from the yang stomach.

In Chinese medicine, organs have important yin-yang counterparts other than the brain. These counterparts must be in balance for health to be maintained. Imbalance leads to eventual disease manifestation. So although the spleen is not considered a digestive organ here in Western medicine, it is crucial in other medicines of the world. The spleen stores the yin energy, the nutrition of the person. Even though it is not considered to produce digestive enzymes, indeed it is a yang function of the stomach, the spleen is necessary for vitality and usefulness of digestive processes. How much disease occurs because the spleen is neglected. We do understand the spleen as a filter for immunity and a storage site for blood, shouldn't it make sense that it be the warehouse for our vitality?

Herbs for spleen support might be mullein (again), blood builders such as alfalfa leaf, bloodroot, and foods such as beets. Again, good nutrition is paramount in spleen support, and super foods such as blackstrap molasses, honey, and kelp may also be quite useful.

CHAPTER 2

Diet

Diet plays an important role in the management of gastrointestinal health which directly impacts nutrition. It is very important here to remember some needs are pretty much required by everybody; but we are unique in our absorption, digestion, and functional capabilities. One remedy that works well for one may not be the best choice for another, although superficially they look good. For example, with a person who has limited digestion, and/or is deficient, raw foods can be weakening. These people need help maintaining temperature, and the work that goes into digesting raw foods is restricting to these people. Not that a deficient person cannot chew an occasional carrot or celery stick, but these cannot be the sole diet recommendations. Nuts are another example of food that can be very difficult to digest. So you must always strive to find what works for you as an individual.

Some may assume or even argue you should eat only that which your body craves. This is untrue, however, as addictions are great examples of foods and beverages our body cannot only readily accept but demand through cravings. Our body, the vehicle we carry ourselves around, should be cared for with thoughtful intent, knowledge of our ability, and patience.

Children most readily accept sugar, which causes all kinds of known health problems when used in excess. Learning which foods and how they might benefit health is an ongoing process, but every gain will likely endure as health overall improves. Healing is a process, and I often tell patients, three steps forward, one step back; two steps forward, two steps back; two steps forward, two steps forward and so on as long as you are moving forward in your overall health, and at least not continuing to move back.

Depending on constitution and environment exposures, we should strive for a diverse diet that is as wholesome and organic as possible. Food sensitivities modify this approach correspondingly. Elimination tests, in which you remove a particular suspected food for three weeks to a month, may give you clues to these sensitivities. The reactions can be measured by laboratory blood work in the form of antibody titers, an immune reaction. These tests do not determine the histamine response but the antibody response. Patch allergy testing relies on a histamine response and is less frequently used. These blood tests are available by physicians who understand alternative or complementary principles. These diets can be very limiting for a time as the body learns to readjust its immune system. It is important to maintain adequate nutrition while following elimination diets. We should pay attention to our intuition and how we feel after the removal of possible sensitivities Acid overproduction is a common symptom of food sensitivity.

Requirements for Good Nutrition

Good nutrition not only includes adequate digestion but adequate and efficient absorption as well as assimilation of nutrients. Digestion occurs when we have the necessary environments and enzymes for optimum breakdown of nutrients. This includes not only normal stomach acid but also adequate enzyme production from the salivary glands, intestinal cells, pancreatic glands, and liver. Normal bile from the liver is also a necessary ingredient for good, adequate digestion. After digestion has been addressed, the cells lining various intestinal regions are important in the uptake of the broken down nutrients. When the intestinal lining is damaged from inflammation or poor digestive processes, these cells not only cannot adequately take in nutrients but also cannot rebuild themselves because their nutrition is weak. When poorly digested and poorly absorbed foods are passed further down where fermentation takes place, toxins and gasses are created. This ultimately weakens vitality further as the stresses build upon themselves.

Lastly, we must have good assimilation of nutrients. Assimilable nutrients are user friendly. This concept is often missed, especially in Western medicine. But certain "nutrients" have very poor nutritional value because they are not brought into the cells requiring them for use, or cannot be effectively used for other reasons. Assimilation is the ability of our body to use the nutrients provided to it. This occurs after the nutrients have been absorbed into the blood.

For example, inorganic calcium such as calcium carbonate is potentially very damaging to our body, and many supplements contain this harmful "nutrient." Calcium carbonate is nothing more than chalk, and our body cannot put this calcium into the nervous, bone, and other vital tissues as it is required. In fact, it may be effective only in scrubbing the bowel. When absorbed this form of calcium floats around in the blood, possibly contributing to deposits in joints, in tendon insertions, along the arterial walls, in the kidneys, etc. Think about it, why is it we take so many supplements with calcium, we drink so much milk? We have the best-fed people in our country, yet we have osteoporosis as a leading cause of health problems, we have kidney stones and bone spurs and, especially, heart disease in the form of hard arteries, which is so extremely common?

What To Do

It is important to figure out what works uniquely for you, keeping in mind getting quality nutrition as much as possible. Here are some recommendations though which improve digestion.

1. Minimize stressful people and situations. Stress is probably the worst environmental risk to a healthy lifestyle, causing damage and impairment from digestion to immune function. Studies constantly are reporting correlations of stressful situations with poor health and serious health risks. Not only does our body work sub-optimally, we tend to make poor choices that further damage our health. People under stressful and negative situations tend to put less priority in taking care of themselves. Do not underestimate the stress in your life, and do what it takes to take control of this with good advice and support. Stop negative environments, including critical people and thinking. Move forward but be very patient with the process. Put boundaries on what you will live with.

2. Chew thoroughly. This was already stated, alkalizing and liquefying your food with saliva is very important to the initiation of digestion. Chewing the food thoroughly also breaks down protein molecules, easing stress on the stomach as well as digestion further down. Remember to drink fluids more between mealtimes to decrease the dilution of the salivary digestive enzymes.

3. Encourage effective digestion with beneficial habits. For example, drink lemon water and /or eat bitter salad greens prior to your meal. Sour and bitter tastes stimulate digestive processes. There are also effective spices that stimulate digestion including cumin and cayenne. Cumin can be added to the main dish while cayenne is traditionally in salsa prior to the meal but could be beneficial in

the main dish as well. This suggests a reason it is traditional for Mexican food to start with salsa dishes.

4. Good food choices. Eat plenty of quality foods including those with valuable essential fatty acids, such as avocados. Feed your body as healthfully as possible, and especially include sources of plant-source minerals and polyunsaturated fresh oils. Nuts such as almonds can be made into an extremely nutritional drink by soaking and slow cooking in pure water. Whole nuts may be a problem for some with bowel inflammation and this should be remembered. Chew nuts well. Nuts in the form of butters and milks are much better absorbed and assimilated. Be sure all oils are fresh. Choose other nutritive foods such as soybeans, celery, dark leafy lettuce, swiss chard, and greens cooked in garlic, olive oil, and carrots as well. Olive oil is great cooking oil and serves much nutritive value. Fresh garlic is certainly protective; you do not necessarily have to take supplements. It does take a little time though cutting up the garlic, but I consider this time well spent; my family is healthy.

Examples of healthful foods for most include but are not limited to foods such as these:

1. Avocados, essential fatty acid foods,
2. Fruits, depending on sensitivities and constitutions,
3. Vegetables, steamed for deficient and weak persons. Chew well for best nutrition. Juiced for super nutrition and fasting purposes, and
4. Whole grains-breads and foods made from gently processed and fresh whole grains can be very nutritious. By allowing the grains to sprout, you make a wonderful source of super food, the most well known probably being wheat grass, although other grains such as barley and alfalfa seeds can be used. Sprouts are very nourishing and strengthening and can benefit those not allergic or sensitized

to the particular grain; the chlorophyll is wonderful and very helpful in building blood.

Many grains have been over processed. Also, grains may become contaminated when not dried or stored properly. Choose grains wisely at the grocery store; choose quality over cost, and read your labels. White bread and white sugar are definitely depleting to you but also grains that have been on the shelf too long or have been improperly stored or prepared. Bake your own bread quite easily with the mixes available at health stores. Many more contemporary grocery stores are more health conscious, and so it is becoming increasingly easier to buy healthier foods if you know what you are looking for. You can buy baking mixes that cost a little more for grains other than wheat, a very common sensitizer. Whoever buys the product determines what kind of food is being made available; if you are a knowledgeable shopper regarding food, the poor quality foods will not sell. And if they do, it is not off your hide or health.

Once in a while a brownie sure is good, but the issue is amount consumed. And even brownies can be made with nutritious ingredients.

5. Another wonderful food is honey. Use maple syrup too as a sweetening agent. Honey is medicinal though; this food is profound in its healing value. There is concern regarding feeding the very young with honey. This is caused by a concern about a risk of botulism, a serious deadly infection. I would concern myself about honey's immunogenecity as well and not use it in the very young for this reason alone. I am not sure of any confirmed cases of botulism, but I may be wrong and have not found them at this point. I would not want to find out by trying this on babies. Honey as a nutritive and restorative for the elderly and deficient individuals may be part of your armamentarium in nourishing

—

deficiencies. You can even apply honey on wounds as a restorative and nutritive and antibacterial agent. Honey has enzymes, polysaccharides, proteins, essential fatty acids, and all kinds of unique products. Honey is excellent as a base for throat lozenges, say with slippery elm, for example. Protect the environment and support the continuation of honeybees.

6. Food combining plays a role in how efficient digestion is. In general, you should not take in sugars with proteins or shortly after protein ingestion. Protein foods require acid more importantly than starches and sugars, so sugars can cause the stomach to prematurely empty for sugar digestion, allowing for putrefaction of poorly digested proteins later on. Your deserts, fruits and similar sweets, should be eaten separately from your protein meals.

Recommended food combinations. Do not eat foods in column one within two hours of column two.

Fruits	Meats
Starches, see exception below	Beans
Sweets	
Juices	
Deserts	

There are exceptions, complex starches (potatoes, spaghetti) tolerate the acid environment of the stomach better than sugars and therefore can be taken in with proteins to a degree. These should generally be eaten earlier in the meal though, to allow them a head start toward the small intestine.

7. Drink ample pure water between meals. This is necessary for adequate detoxification and elimination of wastes. This also promotes saliva formation and flow when mealtime arrives.

—

8. Do not eat too late. The largest meal is usually best in the middle of the day. The last meal should not be of heavy foods and at least three hours before bedtime in most individuals. If you have sugar problems, then a simple snack near bedtime is appropriate but should be limited to a simple sweet potato, rice, or similar food. In Chinese medicine, the liver functions maximally around 11 p.m.; food needs to be ready for processing at this time. Meals eaten late will not be digested in time as well as distract energy from the liver to the digestive tract. Heavy meals have the most distracting energy. Adequately efficient liver function is so important for health. This simple change in diet can be profoundly influential over a period of time.

9. Find out about the source of, including but not limited to, fruits, vegetables, legumes (beans), and grains. Also, seek to prepare them for your needs. For example, if your digestion is weakened, steam your vegetables lightly rather than eat them raw. This is much less work on your digestive system, and you will be able to absorb more of the nutrients. Use as fresh and organic a produce you can get; the next best is quality-frozen vegetables. Do not cook vegetables until they are wilted, but enough to begin starch breakdown. Juicing vegetables is also quite helpful for people with weak digestion. Carrot juice provides a fantastic base for all kinds of nutritive additions such as celery, beets, and parsley. You can get quite a bit of nutrition into your body with simple foods as these. Juicing has been of one of the most tremendous benefits for my own health, and fasting with juices is very common in people who are constitutionally stronger. But for those who are weak, the juice is more an effort at supplying quality nutrition.

Grains and beans are best slow cooked under low heat to preserve nutritional value. These can also make fine beverage milks to drink as is or in shakes, to use in cereals, and can replace the cooking needs supported by dairy milk quite healthfully. The soy and rice milks for example are widely available in many health conscious grocery stores. Also, the milks can be prepared with soy milk makers that are commercially available.

There is commercial need at this present time and in the future for organic fields of beans and grains; the fields should be rotated and nourished with nutrients such as kelp. This is a scary thought for dairy cows. But many more could be more healthfully fed per acre with crops over cattle. Cattle will always have butter, and for deficient individuals, cheese is helpful. But I would not want to be in the red meat industry.

10. Recognize food sensitivities and follow a corresponding diet as best you can. Food sensitization occurs frequently. This is a major cause of pains, swellings, and especially bowel irritation and inflammation. It may take several months to eliminate the reactions to foods you are sensitive too, but the results are worth it if you want to feel well without relying on pharmaceuticals, which do nothing to eliminate the problems causing the pains. Food sensitization occurs when the bowel is swollen, inflamed, irritated, malnourished, or injured by pathogens. The bowel lining becomes leaky, allowing larger molecules to directly enter the bloodstream without liver action. These molecules elicit an immune response that then deposits in various areas, especially distant locations such as joints and tendons. Areas of old injuries often are more prone to food "allergy" reactions.

When the offending foods are eliminated from the diet, the immune response is allowed to soften. This may take several months and even years for some sensitivity. But in general, within a week or two, you will have no doubt if a food is causing your back pain or bowel swelling. When you remove the culprit, these symptoms decrease and eventually go away.

—

11. Avoid harmful foods. These include yeast-risen foods; yeast-derived foods; artificial foods; denatured, devitalized foods such as white flour and white sugar, alcohol, and other intestinal irritants such as pepper and coffee. All of these foods can be particularly damaging and increase symptoms and weaken digestive integrity. Do not underestimate how damaging foods and beverages such as alcohol and pepper alone can be.

Take care of your health to your ability. Read labels. Learn about hazards such as MSG and aluminum. Heavy metals and food additives are increasingly in our diet.

Red meat is also pro-inflammatory and harmful in other ways as well. We would do well to avoid all red meat. Dairy in particular is poorly digested and highly sensitizing, two very undesirable traits that affect most people. Dairy problems affect most of us.

Understand that artificial oils are particularly harmful. These "partially saturated" oils are of an unnatural configuration for assimilation, the necessary function of incorporating a molecule into the body. These oils should be minimized. This goes with rancid oils as well, which are very inflammatory. Never eat old snacks that have a bitter, pungent taste or any other evidence of rancidity. Many prepackaged foods contain partially hydrogenated oils; limit these, especially those of you with gastrointestinal and inflammatory problems.

12. Slow down your eating. Choose restful pleasant surroundings whenever possible. Digestion certainly is impaired when you eat in a hurry or under stressful situations; your body is not sending the circulation where it needs to be for digestion. This allows not only for lining irritation, adding to bowel leaks, but putrefaction by pathogens that get the leftovers in the large intestine. Putrefaction

is a cause of health problems, headaches, and other toxic conditions. This hazard of indigestion can be greatly alleviated and even eliminated through cleansing of putrefactive waste products and proper diet with efficient digestion.

13. Keep the bowels moving. Eat foods that promote bowel regularity. Use gentle medicinal herbs if necessary to restore bowel tone. Constipation certainly aggravates putrefaction. If you suffer from IBD, you certainly may have some partial obstructions throughout the intestinal tract where inflammation has left scarring. In this case, it is especially important to keep the bowels on the loose side to prevent obstruction and a life-threatening situation.

14. Get adequate rest. Simplify your life; make necessary changes to decrease demands that really do not benefit.

About Organic Produce

It is important to support organic produce. Fresh vegetable and fruits of high nutritional value should always be sought. Grains and legumes should be quality as well; we should not be increasing quantity at the expense of quality. The organic food industry needs support and recognition; much better quality food could be provided with better farming standards. People should be willing to pay a little extra for the more healthful food; food choices do play a significant role in medical costs of the future. You are what you eat. Our farmers need our support; but we must expect quality, not over-fertilized, pesticide-exposed, products.

Organic farming can be laborious for credentialing, so sometimes you really need to buy from reputable sources, organic or not. It is not that hard to switch to organic farming techniques, but it does take effort and money. You actually should pull those weeds not spray them. Learn to grow more healthy foods for more health.

We should strive to be an example to the world of health with all our beautiful land, managing it thoughtfully, rather than greedily by pushing it beyond its limits. Our clean water and land is our food supply. We do the same to ourselves with caffeine and other stimulants.

Practicing what you believe in is the best example and influence you can have on any person, group, or country. This begins with how we feed our children, how we manage our homes and families, how we care for our environment and community, and the integrity we bring to our work.

GMO (genetically modified food) is this safe?

GMO foods are of great concern as well. Organic foods can be GMO. GMO refers to genetic modification. The best known example is flounder DNA in corn to allow corn to better weather cooler temperatures. GMO has been used to increase crop yields, protect against insects, and stimulate faster growth. GMO is basically everywhere, unfortunately; and for my family, as best we can, we would avoid GMO food. Food sources do not have to report the food they are providing has been modified genetically; they do not have to disclose this. Soy has unfortunately been one of the victims, as well as corn.

Fortunately, companies can announce the sources are not genetically modified. I would strongly consider these foods safer than foods that have been genetically modified.

Non-GMO is the safer choice if you have one. Hopefully labels will be clear and reputations will be honorable.

In the herbal world, plants living in harsh environments develop substances that help them manage that environment; these substances in turn may determine much of the plants medicinal value. Plants grow specific to regions to serve specific functions in the diet; for example, Texas has a lot of plantain. This plant is nutritive and restorative and would be especially useful to people living here. Rosemary grows well here also, as seen from the above picture. Rosemary is such a valuable medicinal plant.

Some GMO may not be harmful, but how do you know. We certainly have a very ill generation of people and very expensive medical care.

An example of a plant that is most useful under natural living conditions is the great chaparral. Chaparral is a very serious plant for serious disease used by experts only. This plant proliferates in an extremely harsh environment, and this somehow conveys the anti-cancer abilities. These conditions are necessary for Chaparral.

So produce grown in natural conditions with natural soils may be healthier. The body, as well as our environment, does recognize the difference.

CHAPTER 3

Balanced Lifestyle

It is important and beneficial to maintain a structured environment as best as possible where children know what to expect and what is expected of them. The most education we can provide for our children is by our example; and qualities such as patience, responsibility, endurance, peace, forgiveness, and humility go a long way in establishing each of our child's unique identities. Of course, nobody is perfect or will be; but we should make an effort to move forward each day in our spiritual, emotional, and intellectual development. We will always make mistakes, what is important is how we respond to them and the lessons we glean. An encouragement to me is the understanding that we are being transformed daily by the glory of our Lord, each at our own pace and pathway.

Establishing routine and consistency provide our children with a sense of safety and security that nothing else can take the place of. This makes family traditions so vital to our culture, heritage, and identity. For this consistency to be manifest, we have to be aware of our surroundings and the people around us. We must be sensitive to the needs of those around us, especially those dependent on us for their own spiritual, emotional, and physical development.

It is an awesome responsibility and privilege to be given even one child, or a quiver full of children, and this may be our most important contribution to society. Active involvement in the lives and welfare of the young is paramount to the survival of any species. A problem we face though with raising our children is an increasingly rapidly moving society where competitiveness and greed are all too prized. We are bombarded with chaos and confusion from the minute we enter this world, in many cases with constant noises and activity. Much of this is not beneficial; and an important message is to be quiet, slow down, and let the peace surround you. Often we become just too wound up to stop the noise, and we get further and further into habits of busyness and noise.

Starting good dietary habits as early as possible can greatly affect the abilities and opportunities available to our children. Habits only develop with repetition. Repeatedly educate your young about healthy food choices, and especially by your own example and leadership, they will draw to these foods. There is so much deception in foodstuffs with resulting illness, disease, and weakness. Often parents just are not aware of the harmful and possibly harmful substances that are allowed in our commercial foods. This awareness is a primary goal, as there are long-term consequences to poor foodstuffs. It is true that you are what you eat, what else could you be in the physical. Our body is not to be worshipped though; it is only the temple which our spirit resides in. That does not mean we should not attempt to care for our body and learn about its functions. That does not give us license to continue to wallow in ignorance and self-pity, but it encourages us that there are those efforts which will support life available to us if we will seek them.

Avoid toxic exposures as much as possible

It is important as well to be aware of the chemical and toxic exposures in our surroundings, especially in areas where our children frequent

—

often. This is not simply to prevent outright illness but also to encourage maximum function and development. A clear vessel also might be more receptive to the inner prompting of Jesus, as we have discovered in our family. When we are becoming polluted in our bloodstreams by various substances, it affects our thinking and vitality tremendously. Room air filters that are well maintained, avoiding exposure to cigarette and other fumes, and limiting any exposures to chemicals such as off-gassing products from new paint and furniture should all be strongly considered if you want your children to succeed to the best of their ability.

Also, be aware of the chemicals and products you and your family use, especially products used frequently. Learn to watch out for pollutants in our products and minimize exposure to these. It is not necessarily true that all natural products are safe either, so do not make this assumption. Also, realize we cannot possibly know it all and can only do our best. Get your information from knowledgeable persons, and don't let your own lack of awareness blind you to the truth about our environment. Check your sources of information and be reasonable. Great minds can often come in humble packaging.

Some important ingredients I try to avoid are metal exposures such as aluminum, mercury, and others. Aluminum is often used in cookware, foil, many commercial antiperspirants, and packaging materials such as soda cans. This builds up in your tissues, and there is enough evidence to convince me to keep away from this extremely harmful substance. We have found mineral salts for antiperspirants available at health food stores an effective alternative, although we may require more bathes, particularly in the first three or so weeks after switching from aluminum containing antiperspirants. Aluminum can also be found in baking soda, hair and other body products, and other common items. Often, the baked goods in supermarkets use aluminum baking soda as well as boxed baking products. Certainly a small amount would not kill you or even cause significant harm, but when your body is exposed often enough, harm does result in

—

many. Also, there will be those who seem to be healthy despite all their exposures; fortunately or possibly unfortunately, their body has allowed them more leniencies in its management, but possibly this too will catch up with them. There is evidence that heavy metal poisonings such as aluminum may worsen Alzheimer's-type diseases. In addition, aluminum is in most anti-perspirants possible an added factor in the development of breast cancer. Perspiration is a mechanism of detoxification as well as cooling the body.

Mercury exposure, as well as other metals, is related to amalgam tooth fillings. If possible, have these removed by a skillful and knowledgeable dentist, but be sure to not get any more of these placed in your mouth. The evidence is in, in my humble opinion, and my children will never get amalgams and, hopefully with the appropriate care and nourishment, will not require fillings at all. Amalgam fillings are up to 50 percent mercury, which leaks throughout the digestive system and builds up in areas such as the brain and kidneys. Don't do this. Mercury destroys enzyme activity, causing all kinds of possible disease conditions, for example, the cause of "leaky bowel" often seen in our culture.

Copper levels in our body can be elevated from plumbing sources; it is wise to address this possible toxicity. There is an easily evaluated and relatively cheap test that can be obtained from many reputable laboratories. This test requires a small sample of recent hair growth (that which is closest to your scalp, not the ends of long tresses.) This hair sample can be effectively evaluated for various levels of metals, both those required for life and those that can become poisonous and harmful. Although different body tissues can vary from the levels determined from the hair sample, as the hair sample only gives approximations from the levels within the bloodstream, a general idea about mineral and heavy metal status can be suggested. Certain organs such as the kidneys, brain, and liver can harbor significantly higher levels of heavy metals, which cannot be so readily identified. Poor function of these tissues may not occur until late in the

—

process, causing more confusion to the possible long-term effects of heavy metal poisoning. Laboratories for hair analysis are useful to determine deficiencies as well as excesses.

Control the environment your child lives in

Finally, mealtimes can be a very useful time to establish relationships within the family, as well as outside the family. Mealtimes can especially be used to advantage to establish a peaceful and loving atmosphere where each individual is valued and appreciated. It is best to make mealtimes routine and taken in an unhurried fashion. Although this certainly cannot always be achieved, the goal is worthwhile and pays many rewards in the long term with the improved self-esteem and relationships within and among each member of the family. Mealtime can offer an opportunity for fellowship and consistency in routine.

It is wise to monitor the television programs and music your child listens to and watches. We should be very aware of the thoughts and ideas we are exposed to. Remember hear no evil, see no evil, speak no evil. This is a very wise old saying. Watch out for the children; learn to protect your child as much as you possibly can from harmful relationships. Pray regularly that your child or children will be attracted and exposed primarily loving and positive teachers, friends, and role models. Realize it is not such a bad thing when we do have to learn to work with more difficult individuals. It is important to be aware of the friends and relationships your child keeps. Regularly teach your children from an early age the importance of keeping healthy relationships while being a positive example to others. Consider the posters and pictures as well as the music your child focuses on and keep these as positive as realistic.

CHAPTER 4

Inflammation

Inflammation causes pain wherever it is, wherever it goes. Inflammation and irritation can occur in various ways throughout the gastrointestinal tract. These result in poor bowel function as well as integrity. The bowel lining becomes "leaky," allowing for large molecules to pass directly into the blood. This leads to sensitization to foods and further inflammation and sensitivities. Irritating foods, pathological organisms, and food sensitivities all play a role in causing inflammation. But inflammation in itself involves damaging fats; these include rancid oils, partially hydrogenated oils, and especially arachidonic acid, which is most commonly found in red meat.

Fats

Fats are broken down into fatty acids that are then changed into prostaglandins, and there are several types. The damaging natural fatty acids involved in proinflammatory pathways involve arachidonic acid. This acid is preponderant in red meat; I believe this metabolite is tagged

–

to fear. When we have an unhealthy balance of fatty acids, we promote an inflammatory action as well as an acidic condition leading to further toxicity to the human body.

There are very important beneficial fats. Yes, *fats*. Eat those avocados, they are absolutely wonderful for anyone without an allergy to them. The beneficial effects will be noted rather quickly in your skin. There are beneficial and essential fatty acids, the breakdown products of fats, which are triglycerides, three fatty acids attached to a short chain.

*

Unsaturated fatty acids are anti-inflammatory. These oils require refrigeration because they are not hardened with hydrogen molecules. Monounsaturated fatty acids such as olive oil are more stable because the natural hydrogenation is minimal. Partially saturated oils are dangerous; these oils are artificially altered, adding hydrogen molecules to make the oil more stable. Margarine is a prime example, as is shortening. These are very unnatural and damaging, causing inflammation and such problems as arterial damage.

There are basically three essential fatty acids that are fats that cannot be furnished by the human body. These fatty acids are polyunsaturated, thus, have no hydrogen molecules to harden them. They are unstable, as are all unsaturated oils, and should be refrigerated. They must come from a plant source in fresh abundance.

Unsaturated and polyunsaturated fats are necessary for many bodily functions and membranes, and essential fatty acids are necessary for anti-inflammatory pathways. Examples of wonderful when fresh plant oils include borage seed oil, flaxseed oil, black currant oil, cranberry seed oil, and evening primrose oil—all wonderful. *Keep these refrigerated; check for rancidity.* Rancid oils have a sharp bad taste; *do not ingest rancid oils.* Essential fatty acids (EFAs) are extremely important in counteracting

—

inflammation, and valuable bodily resources are used up with inflammatory reactions. These fatty acids are necessary throughout the body, especially areas of high inflammation. In inflammatory bowel disease, we waste a lot of energy from this inflammation, not a fault of our own although we can do things to minimize this wasting.

The brain and nerve cells require especially ample amounts of anti-inflammatory unsaturated fatty acids especially including the EFAs. The natural plant sources of EFAs do require modifications although small, in the liver for most efficient utilization of the fatty acids and nervous system function. Therefore, it is important when there is liver involvement to consider supplementation with fish oils; these EFAs do not require modifications and thus are readily useful to the nervous system for adequate function and health.

Fish oil is an important example to remember. The fish oils must be from safe clean sources. Fish are potentially contaminated from poor water sources, for example, with mercury. The EFAs from fish, omega 3s and others, do not require the liver for further modification into specific fatty acids, docasohexanoic acid and eicosopentanoic acid (DHA and EPA), necessary for nervous system health. Fish oils are a valuable adjunct to help an overextended liver by providing the nutrients without any work.

Fish must be fresh and properly stored more so than other meats. Although nutritious, eating fish may be limited as a reliable source of omega fatty acids in most diets today. Fish oils are damaged with cooking. You can still take your flax or borage alongside. You can take several gel caps with a full glass of warm tea, not necessarily daily. Salmon often has been dyed red and genetically modified to grow seven times faster. I am so sad for this because, otherwise, salmon is a wonderful source of minerals, especially calcium, as well as EFAs and other valuable nutrients. Choose small fish that are not ground feeders such as orange roughy and tilapia. Fish at the end of the food chain have the highest risk of contamination naturally since they are taking in all the other smaller fish and concentrating the contaminants. Bottom feeders such as catfish may also be a problem, but if your water source and food supply to the fish is good, any fish can be an excellent source of nutrition.

To first heal inflammation, be sure you are feeding your body the protection it needs. Fresh foods such as nuts also may be sources of valuable oils. Olive oil is a favorite source of unsaturated anti-inflammatory fatty acids. This oil is stable because it is "monounsaturated," and has powerful medicinal and nutritive power. Canola should be refrigerated to keep the oil more stable. This one is for baking, rotate this oil regularly and check for rancidity. The healthier oils generally are not stable in heat for any prolonged duration.

Inflammation in IBD manifests in many avenues in addition to bowel complaints. Some people suffer from joint and muscle inflammation, some from nerve inflammation, some from glandular inflammation, and others from skin or other organ inflammation. These vary by individuals and exposures, and most vary in the multitude of symptoms. The symptoms can all be improved by quality oils as adjunct therapy over several months for obvious benefit although worth it early on. Herbs also are of use as are nutraceuticals discussed in later a chapter.

Inflammation should be addressed in a number of ways. For example, (1) nutritionally, as with EFAs; (2) allergically, or discovering what is providing the stimulus; (3) immune modification and correction with herbs and removal of offending agents; 4) minimization of damage of any involved tissues; and (5) encouraging proper healing and restoration of tissue function.

Organs that may need specific consideration to control and minimize tissue damage include the heart, the skin, the kidneys, the spleen, the liver, the joints, the nervous system, as well as the gastrointestinal system. Damage in these tissues leads to longstanding problems.

So as you can see, inflammation from the intestinal tract can profoundly affect an individual, in addition to the wasting sufferers experience if not in check nutritionally. Healing of all involved tissues can be promoted with knowledge of herbal and nutritional medicine.

Boswellia, turmeric, meadowsweet, willow bark, and cooked or dried nettle leaf all are highly recommended for their anti-inflammatory properties.

Antiparasitic and anti-yeast herbs and foods can help in alleviating inflammation by removing immune irritation. Antiparasitics include black walnut, wormwood, male fern, turmeric, hyssop, pumpkin seeds, and pomegranate. Anti-yeasts include black walnut, hyssop, garlic, caprylic acid, and probiotics ("good" intestinal bacteria) such as acidophilus.

Symptoms of inflammation include but are not limited too:

Bowel Irritability and Cancer

These spasms react from irritants, inflammation, and other insults. Diet certainly can be stressed here as important for management. There can be quite painful griping pains, usually with diarrhea, especially in earlier disease. Later disease presents with more obstructive symptoms, so diarrhea may not be there, although the griping pain still will.

In literature, studies support findings that anti-inflammatory medicines protect against colon cancer. Although in Western literature they are suggesting the newer anti-inflammatory medications known as COX-2 inhibitors, baby aspirin has also been found to be helpful in the prevention of polyps that become colon cancers over time. Turmeric, a well-known historical Eastern medicinal herb, has had a long history of safety for colon inflammation and, again in studies to date, has been found very effective in the prevention of colon cancer. The studies follow high-risk patients, those who have had colon polyps that are known to later turn into cancer and patients who have already had colon cancers removed.

—

Arthritis

Joint pain is a hallmark of autoimmune disease, and an early manifestation of bowel problems in many individuals. Not all joint pain is the same, however, and you must think about your own risks and history. Joint, tendon, and muscle pain can often result from "leaky bowel." Leaky bowel occur when damage to the lining has allowed larger molecules directly into the blood, stimulating immune reactions; these immune complexes deposit in previously injured regions as well as joint and other tissue regions.

What kind of known exposures have you had?

What environment are you in most of the day?

Do you have food sensitivities? Cravings?

Is there a *yeast* burden?

What is your genetics suggesting?

Are you constipated?

Have you had known injuries?

How is your diet? Do you vary your diet? Do you try healthy alternatives?

All these things play a role in the manifestation of joint pain, tendonitis, enthesopathy (inflammation at the site of tendon insertions into muscles and bones), and fibromyalgia. There are actually different causes, sometimes overlapping. But joint pain that comes and goes, or doesn't, is certainly a hallmark of an inflammatory response.

An important thing to know about joint inflammation though is that when the joints and tendons are inflamed, for whatever reason, they are especially at risk for trauma. They are swollen and not circulating well. Therefore the inflammation not appropriately considered certainly may become progressive and will in many cases just from minor traumas while the ligaments are inflamed. Also in this regard, it is important to remember that trauma should be allowed adequate healing time, rest, and nutrition to help thwart an inflammatory deposit in the future.

Vascular Disease

It is increasingly recognized the role inflammation plays in causing damage to the inner lining of the blood vessels, heart, kidneys, and other tissues. Indeed, controlling inflammation plays a serious role in the prevention of many common diseases including heart disease. It is common, for example, to take a baby aspirin a day in part of the Western management of heart disease.

Skin Lesions

All kinds of skin changes can occur in patients with inflammatory bowel. These include inflammatory reactions such as rashes and bumps, non-healing or poorly healing wounds, and acne-like bumps that do not respond to conventional acne therapy. These can be quite disfiguring in some, not such a problem in others. Some of these lesions can be painful. When you maximize nutrition and control inflammation with supplements and foods particularly rich in EFAs, you will do much to improve the skin condition. Many topical medicines may help, but nothing compares to internal cleansing and nutrition for skin health.

Kelp is very helpful, taken internally for skin health. Kelp has a large iodine content, so it can cause a rash in some. I am not sure whether the rash is an allergy or a result of a healing crisis. A healing crisis occurs when the body is trying to eliminate too many toxins too rapidly. You can encourage the crisis to end by improving circulation, encouraging sweating, and the function of other organs of elimination, including the lungs, the bowels, the kidneys, and the liver. The skin is the largest organ of elimination by sweating, so drink plenty of fluids and take hot baths frequently. Do not, however, allow yourself to become dehydrated, which would counteract any elimination attempts. The rash can get worse before better as toxins get released. Be sure to stay on a wholesome diet to avoid putting into your body any more toxic load.

Remember, the skin is the outward manifestation of what is going on inside. The bloodstream must be healthy and clean to have healthy skin. The liver also must be functioning well to clear toxins and waste. The bowels need regular movements daily as well to avoid putrefaction and autointoxication that allow toxins into the blood and place more work on the liver.

Juices in particular can help skin conditions. They stimulate bowel motility, and they give fluids and super nutrition and require very little work to digest. With carrot juice, the base for most of my other ingredients (parsley, beets, celery), you may get a little orange with heavy and frequent use, and carrot juice is a wonderful healer. You are not getting vitamin A, you are getting beta-carotene. There is a *big* difference. The liver modifies beta-carotene to vitamin A; you will not get an overdose of vitamin A, the active form, by eating or drinking carrots. The orange from carrot juice is not harmful but probably lets you know you are getting enough. I was so deficient it took me years to develop any orange tint from beta-carotene at all. This orange is only noticeable on my palms and soles. Beta-carotene is the safe form of vitamin A and should not be confused as being the same as vitamin A, which can be harmful if ingested to excess.

Another important thing to realize and accept is the frustration and stress any chronic illness puts on the sufferer and her or his family. You must not give up the hope for a better tomorrow and not take today for granted. There is so much ignorance with inflammatory bowel disease that usually has its most obvious onset during the prime of a person's life.

Survivors are not weak or anorexic but must find foods and habits that work for them, then work together and share their experiences for better understanding. If anything, to survive and maintain a functional life in the midst of a serious illness makes a person strong. Do not allow any person, doctor, friend, or otherwise to tell you not to take care of yourself and do your own homework. Trust yourself. They cannot completely understand what you are facing in your uniqueness. On the other hand, do not let worry, anxiety, and frustration ruin your hope. Learn to understand your thoughts and emotions; do not let them control you. Get adequate rest and freely forgive yourself and others. This will help your mental outlook tremendously. If necessary, get help for these frustrating emotions but realize they are normal for anyone with normal reactions. You have to be above normal to handle the frustration of chronic illness, but do not give in. You certainly can be above normal.

CHAPTER 5

Organ Systems Review

It might be helpful to review the basic organ systems structure and function to better understand disease processes. This may be a review, but there are still points to be sure to understand for better health. I have started from the head to the toes for continuity, but obviously many systems overlap in many uncomplicated as well as complicated ways.

In addition, certain systems should be better understand than the general public is aware of because the future of disease management lies more and more on the patient and the patient's guardians. We will always rely on Western medicine advances and can have an attitude of gratitude at the possibilities. But we must be more responsible, as we find possible, in protecting and maintaining our own health. Disease can require many healers in managing the manifestations and symptom complexes, but by working together, we can hope for a better outcome as studies are showing. In a current issue, a study showed that those who drank more soy-based products and less dairy were healthier in a number of ways, especially involving the heart function. It is my sincere effort not to cause conflict with your doctor, but find a doctor who can respect your willingness to help solve the cause and problems. I have found few doctors in my particular area who understand the complexity of this approach, but they are becoming more open to the ideas as they see the benefits.

So we will review and consider the value of certain organ system networks and how they may tie into disease evolution, and healing.

1. Nervous system, the God-made "Internet"

Of course, the brain is the most central component to our nervous system with the ability to understand, to process information, and to regulate basic and complex routine bodily functions. It all starts here. In the center of the brain are two glands, the pituitary and hypothalamus, particularly important in regulating hormone activity. Also, there is a gland very deep to the eyes called the pineal gland; this gland is more developed in animals. The pineal is especially sensitive to natural rhythms of the body, for example, primarily melatonin. When sunlight enters our eyes for a certain period of time, the pineal reacts. Each side of the brain store information on movement and memory, depending on location. The front region of the brain focuses on emotions, the sides on hearing, and the very back on vision. In the very center, deep region of the brain, all these messages are transmitted to appropriate regions for activity or inactivity, depending on the message.

Then you have the spinal cord and the generally tapering widths and lengths of various nervous system elements, especially axons extending from nerve bodies, throughout the body to every area and organ in the body to some degree. Some areas are highly innervated, for example, our face, our hands, and very central areas. Our feet are interesting, especially from the perspective of reflexology, and all of the organ healing you can do with gentle and purposeful reflexology of your feet. The hands are also a possible source of therapeutic reflexology. This is a lot of what the art of acupressure and acupuncture is about. Acupressure and acupuncture term these regions as meridians and pressure points. They are basically nervous interconnections that allow the energy of the body, the "chi," to freely flow through the body without blockages. The chi refers more to Oriental medicine, but understanding this, it becomes especially important to remember and study massage as well as reflexology. It is not only muscles and joints that need attention. Study the meridian acupressure points; this can especially support healthy nervous system function.

The nervous system is dependent on our diet for most of its supplies via the bloodstream. Essential fatty acids, minerals, vitamins, and balanced protein are all necessary for nervous system activity. The nervous systems' primary energy source is glucose, which can be directly supplied by eating sugary substances; this overloads not only the nervous system but also other organs such as the pancreas. White sugar and starch products also cost the nervous system and other parts of the body minerals to activate the cells that have taken in the sugar. This is one of the major reasons it is necessary to get sugar in a wholesome form, the minerals are more available with the sugar of carrots, cherries, and apples for example.

Nervous tissue is also more vulnerable to toxicities; levels of toxins such as lead and aluminum tend to accumulate in brain tissue. It is easier for these to get in, than out of the nervous system. I strongly suspect peripheral neuropathies, pains, numbness, and weakness might all be at least contributed to by toxin build up. In addition, body mineral depletion must play a role in the deterioration of the nervous system.

So when we allow our children sugar too often, they become nervous, agitated, and attention deficient. Also, sugary foods causes the body to over-respond to insulin from the pancreas in many children, leading to later causes of low blood sugar, causing further cravings for sweets.

Sugar also freely feeds yeasts, and yeast overgrowth is a severe problem in our children today. Yeasts can cause a variety of symptoms and will be addressed later in the parasite section, to which I believe they belong. A mother can pass yeast overgrowth to her child at birth, especially in a vaginal birth, so a child literally can be born with a yeast overgrowth problem. This should not be taken lightly. Although a relatively small number of yeasts are normal inhabitants, by allowing them to over-proliferate, you set up problems if not now then later.

To help improve the nervous system function, eat plenty of vegetables lightly steamed for best digestion. Also consider supplementing your child with kelp or blackstrap molasses, both are loaded with minerals. Kelp probably must be encapsulated; it is not that tasty to most children. Sneak some in their meal. Fresh nuts contain valuable essential fatty acids. My favorite source of essential fatty acids is avocado. Make your child take a bite whenever possible, for example, in their salad at dinnertime. There are also supplements that support essential fatty acids, among these include flaxseed oil, borage seed oil, evening primrose oil, and black currant oil.

Calcium is important everywhere, especially to the nervous system. Celery sticks are usually readily convincing to eat. These are loaded with absorbable, assimilable nutrients, especially calcium. Carrots and dark green leafy vegetables also have significant, ideal calcium. Do not rely on milk for the sole calcium solution.

Many different substances and chemicals pass around the body, especially via the nervous and circulatory systems. The lymphatic system is also highly responsible in moving fluids and substances of various types. These systems are obviously dependent upon each other for support.

2. Cardiovascular System (Heart and Blood Vessels)

The River of Life

The cardiovascular consists of the heart, the pump, and all of the vessels and tapering capillaries allowing for the exchange of oxygen, as well as nutrients and the elimination of substances. The vascular system

—

is responsible for the delivery of the basic elements to the corresponding tissues. The capillaries in the kidneys are very important therefore and modified specifically for removal of toxins and water management.

Pure fluids and vital foods and nutrients support the healing and regeneration of spent and damaged cells that line the vascular structures.

The heart consists of layers, the endothelium most in the inside, the muscular layer, the myocardium, and pericardium, the outermost layer, which actually is a sac of fluid to minimize friction from an active heart. So heart disease can manifest internally with inflammation in the inner lining (endothelium) or could involve the outermost or middle layers of heart tissue, different disease processes ensue although symptoms may be similar.

To support a healthy heart, strictly minimize red meat, partially hydrogenated oil, and saturated fats of animal origin. These fats are very harmful, especially to the endothelium that is most exposed to blood. Rancid oils are also a serious health threat with aflatoxin one of the resulting toxicity problems. Start this as soon as you understand why you should understand the activity and qualities of different oils. Supplement yourself with essential fatty acids, especially omega-6 and—6s of the polyunsaturated linoleic, linolenic, and oleic (C9), which are all healthful. Avocadoes and olive oil are very heart-friendly fats.

From as early as possible, the heart should be fed well. The heart is exposed to all the blood as it propels the blood throughout the body via vessels of varying sizes. After receiving blood from throughout the body, the heart takes the more toxic blood with waste products from the liver and other areas to the heart to be sent through the lungs. The lungs are responsible for clearing the waste products of cells, especially carbon dioxide (CO_2). The blood returns to the heart for propulsion again throughout the body to continue supplying fresh supplies and removing wastes with the help of the liver, kidneys, lungs and skin.

As you can understand, the heart is exposed to a lot of things that get into the blood. Bacteria can involve the heart through a thorough tooth cleaning, causing problems for some. It is regular practice for any individuals with heart disease to get antibiotics before and after dental cleaning. Anything riding around in the blood vessels affects this system. The inner lining of blood vessels can also be irritated by certain exposures. For example, it is well accepted that caffeine is hard on the heart. Other toxins such as fumes and other airborne pollutants, such as cigarette smoke, also damage the inner lining of the heart.

The blood vessels also have developed their own set of problems. Varicose veins and spider veins are a nuisance and can even become painful and severe. Varicosities occur at areas of venous strain. This is usually when the blood has been more stagnant. Veins are unique; they have one-way valves that allow them to push blood upward by the muscles around them. When these valves become damaged, they can allow for more stagnation. So elevating tired legs does have its advantages.

Healthful food is important to all the heart disease today. Unfortunately, many with heart disease find out late in the process when it is more difficult and takes more diligence and patience to see improvement. Keeping the blood as pure as possible, supplying an abundance of beneficial nutrients such as blueberries and raspberries can do so much in preventing heart and vascular disease. The eyes have tiny vessels that vision depends on; by keeping vessels healthy and flexible with the right nutrients, these will protect vision as the years go by.

Flavanoids are also very nutritious to vascular tissue, and berries of all kinds are especially nourishing to heart and vessel tissue. They protect in several ways including anti-oxidation.

Garlic is especially heart friendly as well among many of the plants with wonderful virtues.

Fish can be very nourishing to the heart with the omega-3 essential fatty acids readily available for nervous system use. You have to eat fresh and well-cooked fish from reputable sources.

Every organ has small capillaries that allow for the transfer of the substances relative to the specific function. Coenzyme Q10 is very useful at these capillary interchanges, with much energy being consumed. The blood goes throughout the body allowing each organ to perform their specific duties.

To help prevent hardening of the arteries, calcification of the arterial wall, you must continue to encourage your family to drink plenty of fresh and pure water, get regular exercise, and watch your calcium supply. If you get calcium from blackstrap molasses, celery, dark green leafy vegetables you will benefit from both absorbable as well as assimilable calcium and other minerals. Never use supplements with calcium carbonate as their source of calcium. Read you labels. Calcium carbonate is everywhere, and is often touted on foods as a good source of calcium. This form of calcium is poorly assimilated, if at all judging by the amount of osteoporosis in our country. Dairy also does not have a very useful supply of calcium, dairy wastes a lot of calcium in the kidneys with its high phosphate and protein level. Theses poorly assimilated calcium either must be excreted, either by not absorbing or via the kidneys. This puts extra demands on the kidneys promoting stone formation ultimately. The delicate kidney tubules are even more vulnerable to some toxins than the heart, because they must deal with so much waste.

Try to get your child to get used to these healthy foods early but remember all ages need these foods. Avocadoes are also especially heart friendly. Berries are extremely nourishing to the lining of blood vessels, so always indulge your children to berries. Grapes are also especially heart healthy.

If you are concerned about cholesterol consider herbs such as garlic. Garlic has wonderful properties including lowering cholesterol. Cholesterol control ultimately requires good liver work to keep the bloodstream clean. Soy contributes in many. Learn to enjoy soy foods such as milk. Provide soy for your family. After two weeks of soymilk, you will adjust to it's flavor. Almond milk also contains quality unsaturated fatty acids for good circulation. There is a precaution in that many of these fortified milks contain calcium carbonate, a lesser value calcium form.

For heart health drink plenty of pure water and indulge in red raspberry leaf tea. Hawthorn is very helpful over long-term periods to help build up a weakened or damaged heart, so use hawthorn berry faithfully for a long period of time to help strengthen the heart. Hawthorn berry is very safe. Elderly people with potentially more sensitivities especially should start herbals such as hawthorn gently. Over time those on heart medications may find themselves needing to lower the dose as the heart responds more effectively. There may be rare allergy not reported, but I have seen a fixed rash that goes away after stopping the herb. It looks like a cluster of tiny blood vessels in a small location on the skin.

Exercise is very important for heart health. Not only does exercise increase heart strength, it allows for more sweating and cleansing, getting the blood to go throughout the body. Exercise is moving the blood. This reminds of an old Chinese saying, "Where the chi goes, the blood follows." Get moving around and let the chi and blood flow freely.

Another profound heart remedy is cayenne. This powerful herb can get someone from a shock state and can be especially useful to the elderly rather than children (especially heart attack cases). But a small amount of cayenne in a child as remedy for any heart weakness should be considered. Cayenne should be in every medicine chest as not only does it support circulation but it also may stop bleeding depending on the size of the hemorrhage. Small doses of cayenne are quite potent.

3. The Respiratory System

The nose, the air passageway (pharynx), and lungs generally comprise our respiratory system. Many authorities also consider the skin our third lung, which I can understand why. Our skin with its pores can help eliminate a lot of toxins, especially in warm water followed by dry brushing gently. Some oxygen also is taken up by the skin, but not enough obviously. Treatment through the skin is a valuable approach to decreasing the load of toxic exposures. Consider a warm bath with plenty of hot tea sweetened to taste, preferably honey. Do not let yourself get dehydrated, but sweating out toxins has a very long history.

The lungs work directly with the heart to oxygenate the blood while allowing the escape of carbon dioxide (CO_2). There are tiny vessels that allow the exchange to take place as the blood passes through the lungs. Our lungs can be very vulnerable to outside conditions. Breathing through the nose can help to protect the lungs, as the nasal turbinates help to filter and warm the entering air, required for the exchange in the lungs. Also, regular deep breathing can do wonders for relaxation in a quiet setting. Deep breathing helps lung function. Deep breathing helps to expand the deep recesses of your lungs. Lungs sometimes become scarred or partially collapsed especially in older people. Practice and encourage appropriate breathing. Especially heed warnings about smoking. In children, discuss the severe addiction potential as they will not worry so much about their future lungs and will think they are invincible.

4. The Glands

From top to bottom, the glands include both active and passive functions depending on their unique qualities.

Historically, glands included not only the glands that secrete specific hormones, such as the thyroid, but also included the lymphatic tissues. Starting from the top, you have the tonsils and adenoids, the lymphatics in the back of your throat. These are connected by a lymphatic network similar to the neighboring the bloodstream vessels. The lymphatics are necessary for screening and filtering what comes inside you. The lymphatics have multiple lymph nodes along their path that allows stronger filtration as pathogens and wastes are sorted. The lymphatics move down all around the neck to and down throughout the body, especially in the trunk of the body. There are lymph nodes throughout your body for immune surveillance.

The appendix is a valuable gland; keep this at all costs by watching your diet and the amount of mucus food (breads) you eat.

Sometimes nodes can calcify and feel hard. This is not necessarily a problem unless the nodes become large and/or painful. Large painless nodes also need evaluation. You must get a physician involved to determine the cause for many of these.

Secretory glands

Glands secrete many important substances to help support life and well being by responding to the environment. These substances include hormones, such as growth hormone, cortisol, epinephrine, melatonin, and thyroid hormone. The list is continuously added to as we discover more about ourselves and the various messengers in our bodies.

There are also local factors that allow for internal communication, such as prostaglandins and catechins. Individual cells produce these substances as opposed to glands. We are becoming more aware of the various interplays between the messenger systems. The glands though are extremely important in regulating body responses and functions.

The pituitary gland at the top is the master gland, sending most of its messages to the hypothalamus. This is an important gland that controls many automatic bodily functions, as well as responses to the environment. The hypothalamus regulates and further delivers the message to the specific gland for a specific activity. The hypothalamus is extremely, closely tied to the pituitary; nothing involves one without somehow directly involving

—

the other. Then you have kind of a small, inconspicuous pineal gland, developed variously in different species. The pineal deals with rhythms of the body, well known for managing the sleep/wake cycle (melatonin). The pineal also is very close in relationship to the pituitary but not quite as directly as the hypothalamus. The pineal responds to sunlight exposure from incoming messages from our eyes. This is why light therapy can be beneficial when done appropriately.

Other glands include the *thyroid*, necessary for metabolism, and the *parathyroids* (usually four) that regulate calcium metabolism. Kelp is very supportive to these glands, particularly the thyroid. The thyroid is a difficult gland to assess; many have thyroid problems and a lot more may not even be aware there is a problem. If your metabolism or energy and appetite are low, consider the thyroid. If you get palpitations or panic attacks, consider a malfunctioning thyroid. Keep your children away from too much fluoride in toothpaste and tap water loaded with chlorine. If they are swimmers, supplement them with a lot of blood cleansers. Support their liver more diligently because of their added toxin exposure, so consider kelp.

The *thymus* gland is important for immune function and efficiency. This gland degenerates with age but should be respected more than it is. The gland lies just under the sternum at the neck hollow. Most of the gland's work seems to be done before birth, but I wouldn't doubt it didn't have a subtle influence now.

Sitting on top of your kidneys, included in your back are two *adrenal glands*. These glands are poorly appreciated in Western medicine until they are completely failing. Chronic fatigue is one possibility when the adrenals are failing their activity. Adrenal glands are important for managing mineral content with the support of the kidneys, as well as for managing stress in any form by providing stress hormones such as cortisol. Cortisol is importance for managing the physical stress response. If you have been under stress, physical and/or mental, your adrenals likely are on high demand. If you are moving to another area and your child is having trouble with the transition, support adrenal function. Peas and fresh green beans especially support adrenal health. Licorice root in small daily doses can also be extremely useful in supporting or encouraging adrenal health.

Our *testes* and *ovaries* are also extremely important glands. They are not only responsible for the sex characteristic features but also in reproduction itself. Good diet and a pure bloodstream will benefit these glands to function efficiently as well as allow for healthy reproduction. Black cohosh, mullein, nettle, and red raspberry all support these glands. Also, keep electrical gadgets away from this area. Too often I see people, including kids, with cell phones attached to their waist. This to me is asking for trouble in time.

Males have an organ unique to them (our counterpart being the uterus)—the *prostate* gland. It is ever important to respect and watch out for this gland, for it can become layered with calcium deposits, causing morbidity and even cancer in some. The prostate is mostly responsible for sperm travel and nourishment, but surely, there are other poorly understood prostate functions. The gland is somewhat encased in a protective layering of tissues, so getting circulation to the area can be a significant problem. Nevertheless, the gland can be protected with good eating and sexual habits. Germs can assuredly get caught in the prostate to cause misery like no other. Regularly voiding and safe sexual practices may help decrease the risk.

Teach your kids their worth and love them unconditionally, help them to show love in appropriate ways by educating them by words as well as example. Also, provide the most secure and routine environment, especially when your children are young, but also as they pass through their teens. Again, educate, educate, educate. Teach self-esteem early as well as appropriate love expression. Don't only think females have self-esteem issues; be very aware of your child's world at all ages.

For prostate as well as all urinary health drink plenty of fluids including cranberry as it benefits the renal linings. Cranberry juice alkalinizes, which is healthful, and the juice actually prevents the bacteria or other organisms from clinging on to the lining. I particularly recommend gravel root for any calcium deposits, including in the prostate. Mullein tea also benefits this, as any, gland. The tea may be drunk or used as a compress, depending on intention. You of course may do both. Also, drink plenty of nettle tea along with other healthful fluids. Marshmallow herb is the favorite renal remedy in our home.

Breast diseases tend to occur in females, but males are increasingly getting problems. Breast health is of prime concern for any woman, every woman has concern, and childless woman may be even at more risk. Family history is important but not always present. It is important to know your body. Checking yourself after menstrual cycles and regularly as well as routine mammograms are important. I follow mammograms to not see cancer, I am not looking to see cancer, but see it is not there. As much as one in eight women get breast cancer, and odds increase with advancing age.

Minimize or even stop using aluminum-based antiperspirants. Detoxify yourself of aluminum and use natural crystal deodorant or other natural deodorant that works for you. I firmly believe the aluminum may block up important pores for detoxification. Watch out for aluminum, it is everywhere, in baked goods and on bake-ware as well. Baking powder may contain aluminum (usually does), read labels. Watch out for aluminum in the bakery. Read labels. Take regular warm bathes while drinking plenty of healthful tea to prevent dehydration. Sweating is helpful for any detoxification program.

Breasts also benefit from a vegetarian or vegan diet. Especially the exclusion of red meat has proven itself to have protective possibilities by minimizing arachidonic acid, a potent inflammatory agent. Eating abundant nutritious foods and including essential fatty acids are essential to breast and overall health. Herbals such as mullein are good for breast health. Take an active role in prevention and early detection of this dreaded problem which has afflicted so many. Check yourself and teach your children the habit of routinely checking for any evidence of a "rock." Breast lumps that are more suspicious for cancer feel very firm like a rock, Breast cancer continues to affect younger and more patients. Seek experienced and professional help when dealing with breast cancer or the possibility of cancer. And again, because of the high odds, check your mammograms.

Exercise promotes breast health in general. Keeping the circulation moving vibrantly on a regular basis can stimulate healing and further vitality by strengthening muscle. Allowing yourself to sweat on a regular basis is good for purification.

Medicinal oils and herbal poultices and compresses offer promise to breast problems. Plantain could help to pull out necrotic tissue while stimulating healing. Keep the liver healthy, and the breasts are somewhat more protected. But remember breast disease may be a very random disease.

The *spleen* could also be categorized as a glandular tissue, a very large reservoir and filter. This gland is very important in the storage of immune and nutrient properties. The blood slowly filters through this gland, allowing for the removal of waste and debris.

The spleen is highly valued in Chinese medicine, being a cornerstone of health. Western medicine has yet to realize the importance of spleen health with a healthy diet. Spleen contains vitality. In Chinese medicine, the spleen is the yin of the stomach's yang. Spleen has storage properties, the stomach, fiery digestive properties.

Lastly, the *pancreas* is a very busy gland. It has functions in both helping with digestion as well as control of blood sugar levels, termed exocrine and endocrine functions. Different glands throughout the pancreas have specific functions. Thus the pancreas is actually an island of glands. The endocrine glands secrete insulin into the blood; the exocrine glands secrete digestive enzymes through the pancreatic duct directly into the duodenum, the first portion of the small intestine.

—

5. Our Structural System

Collagen and bone make up our structure that allows us to be "packaged" as well as to move about. Collagen is everywhere in our body, providing the substance for holding tissues together and allowing for movement. Elastic fibers are also very important, especially to the skin as we age, it seems; but it is also protective for your child to be limber. Minerals again are important in maintaining all of our structure as well as in supporting its rapid growth. It is so important to get your child to eat healthy calcium and other mineral sources early in life; they grow so fast. Blackstrap molasses is a powerful bone-building substance. Exercise also helps to strengthen bone as well as improve flexibility. Essential fatty acids are also important for this system, especially the skin.

6. Digestion

Digestion is the cornerstone of health. This includes the mouth with well taken care of teeth, the esophagus that leads the food to the stomach. The stomach secretes hydrochloric acid, especially necessary to break down protein but also important for protection from parasite entry. After the food passes out of the stomach, it enters the small intestine, consisting of three parts. The duodenum is relatively short and is most responsible for secreting digestive enzymes. The liver and pancreas also secrete digestive enzymes and substances (bile to break up fat) into the duodenum. This is where the gallbladder enters. After the duodenum has efficiently broken down nutrients, the remainder of the small intestine including the jejunum and the ileum absorbs the nutrients. Vitamin B12 is absorbed toward the end of the small intestine in the ileum with the help of a substance provided for by the stomach, intrinsic factor (IF). If the stomach is not secreting adequate IF then there is risk of vitamin B12 deficiency. This problem does occur, and vitamin B12 is available at health food stores in under the tongue preparations for direct absorption into the blood. Some older family doctors also give B12 shots, which do seem to improve the energy of the patient. All the B vitamins should be attended to for healthy metabolism; it is just B12 that needs a little help in getting absorbed. And with our mucus-filled diet and manipulation of stomach functions, it is not surprising.

The liver should also be included in the digestive system although like others, it performs a multitude of other functions not only digestive. The liver is a storehouse, a filter, and most importantly, a detoxifier. There are at least three phases of detoxification, and the liver is responsible for these pathways. The liver must be functioning properly to adequately secrete bile to break up fats, exposing nutrients. The liver also forms many important blood constituents, such as clotting factors.

The liver stores sugar in a readily obtainable form for responses from the adrenals, epinephrine, sent to increase the blood sugar level when low. Excess ingestion of sugar can be put here, or the liver can modify proteins and ketones for sugar. The liver also makes other necessary enzymes and proteins while providing a filtering system for incoming foods as well as blood constituents and wastes. The liver has areas where the immune cells sit by the flow of blood, easily reaching for the contaminants. These cells are termed kupfer cells.

The liver has an amazing ability to regenerate itself, thus allowing for such a degree of alcoholism in our country as well as others. The liver can sustain quite a bit of abuse. Symptoms slowly increase, and ill health takes on. The liver should be exposed to clean water and air, pure wholesome food, and a gentle diet. In delicate or susceptible individuals, the liver should be supported regularly through detoxifying and regeneration.

Garlic, milk thistle, barberry, and dandelion are favorite liver remedies. Again, drink plenty of fluids. For acute toxin exposure, MSM (methylsulfonymethane), a supplement, and alpha-lipoic acid both have qualities that support phase 2 detoxification. Along with milk-thistle,

—

these supplements help to protect the liver from the byproducts of phase 1 detoxification, often the cause of liver toxicity and damage (next to alcoholism and poisonings). The phase 1 (best example is cytochrome P450) is over-stimulated, leading to an overload on sulfation, phase 2. Phase three is for substances the other phases cannot adequately solubilize, everything else. There are basically three main methods of detoxification: (1) conjugation, (2) sulfation, and (3) attaching other moieties to allow solubility.

Bile is very important for the absorption of fats. Essential fatty acids are taken in with bile. Bile also is a method of excretion, as much of the bile is evacuated. Bile darkens stool. Light stools can suggest poor biliary flow. Floating stools suggest poor fat digestion. All this requires some liver care. Herbs such as barberry and bitter foods such as mixed salad greens stimulate liver function. Lemon in water prior to a meal can also help liver function as well as salivation. Salivation is important to digestion while it alkalinizes. Alkalinizing wholesome diets keep you and your children healthy. Cancer doesn't hang around alkalinity. This does not mean you should go eat a box of baking soda, but you certainly can soak in Epsom salts for purification and alkalinization.

The appendix usually attaches to the last part of the ileum, possibly performing immune surveillance. Then the food passes into the colon. It is here that water and minerals and necessary bile are absorbed. Cancer must be contributed by toxic wastes stored throughout the intestine, especially if stagnant and persistent. Teach your children to go to the bathroom when they need to, try to learn not to wait and wait and wait. This is very harmful to the colon in particular. We get less responsive to the urge, and eventually, constipation is a problem. Some always have the problem, and must consider proper foods to assist this more rapidly. Minimize the absorption of toxins by regularity. As well as yourself, have your children go to the bathroom on a regular basis, sometimes even though she or he may not need to at the time. Have them at least try on a regular basis to help prevent them from holding in for convenience.

7. Genitourinary System

Keeping this system healthy sometimes does not take a lot of active work, but unfortunately, some of our children as well as us, are more prone to urinary problems. Kidney stones are the result of years of calcification that begin in early life, possibly. The renal system is intricately involved with the adrenal glands, which sit on top of the kidney. One adrenal sits on each kidney sending many messages yet to be identified as these two organs interact. The GU system includes the kidneys, the ureters, the bladder, the urethra, the prostate, the vagina, the penis, the scrotum, the urinary opening, and the tissue around this area, the perineum. Keeping this system healthy can start early like everything else. Minimize exposure to carbonated beverages and keep the amount of protein at a healthy balance. Support healthy kidneys with ample juice, such as grape and orange. There are many herbs than can help the renal system function but protecting against damage in the first place, again limiting exposures to toxins that damage delicate kidney tubules, is the best medicine.

CHAPTER 6

Liver Health

Our liver is a tremendously important organ that is very resistant to damage and with a strong ability to heal itself and regrow tissue. This organ is primarily responsible for filtering the blood, especially as it returns from the gastrointestinal tract; so when toxins are absorbed, the liver is the first place they go. The liver is also extremely important in producing factors necessary in the bloodstream for immune function and coagulation, having much effect on circulation. Our liver is necessary for hormone modulation and breakdown as well as fat and sugar storage and breakdown. Free radicals are charges released from damaged cells and waste products; they damage cell membranes by floating freely and attaching to various tissue surfaces.

The liver has a tremendous purpose in free radical scavenging (collecting these damaging charges.) This is one of the primary means the liver removes toxins, with the enzyme called glutathione peroxidase among other mechanisms.

We understand our liver in terms of infectious processes, genetic processes, alcohol and other medication damage, and elevated cholesterol with its implications and pharmaceutical medications. In Western medicine, we use a small assortment of liver enzymes in the bloodstream to determine if the liver is undergoing any damage. These may be unreliable in patients though to determine toxicity, unless very severe. When the liver is full of toxins, it does not necessarily release enzymes into the blood. These enzymes are released in response to cellular injury with release of its internal contents. If the cells do not leak out its contents, laboratory enzyme levels may be normal. Also, cholesterol can provide a clue to the function of the liver although a high level can be significant for poor liver breakdown of cholesterol; an extremely low level may be present in patients who are malnourished from liver disease. Severe alcoholics, for example, often have low cholesterol levels, 100 or so. These low levels may also be an indicator of poor liver function. Triglycerides also may indicate liver function, with very high levels being associated with liver toxicity. Levels greater than 750 or so have a high risk of pancreatitis as a result. Pancreatitis is a very painful and potentially deadly complication of liver disease and especially of very high fat levels that have resulted from liver disease.

Pharmaceutical medications used in an effort to lower cholesterol and/ or triglyceride levels may be necessary but also harmful to liver function. Although I do not recommend going off these abruptly, I recommend working on and clearing your liver to decrease the requirements for these strong, sometimes costly medications. Consider minimizing or even avoiding medications that are known to be damaging to the liver, such as acetaminophen and certain antibiotics and antifungals. Use these only when necessary and keep their dosages to a minimum. Like I said, the liver has a remarkable ability to recover, but you still must respect this organ.

The Best Time To Eat

According to the Chinese clock, the liver maximally functions between 11:00 and 1:00 a.m. or roughly at this time. It is recommended that no new foods be ingested at this time, as the liver now is both busily assimilating nutrients and detoxifying various products of ingestion, inhalation, and metabolism. The liver is thought to perform minimally twelve hours later for these purposes, so taking in meals at noon is probably a good idea or close to noon. Probably the largest meal is best consumed at this time. Many highly respected and gifted healers will agree that a modest simple meal of complex carbohydrates such as those in brown rice, oats, or sweet potatoes is well tolerated at the evening meal or if blood sugar levels are at risk. Take your more complex meal earlier, so the nutrients are available to be assimilated well as liver function increases in function to peak function again at 11:00 p.m. Your nighttime snack, if you require one, should be simple and nourishing and especially digestible with little energy requirements although it must not the heavily processed poor food value items we have so readily available.

Liver Functions

1. Assimilate nutrients
2. Build proteins
3. Filter blood
4. Involve multiple immune functions
5. Detoxify chemicals and waste products

The liver has amazing regenerative capacity and also has the storage ability for various nutrients (such as glycogen) as well as toxic substances. Fat tissue is one major means our body uses to store unnecessary chemical products; thus, a fatty liver is seen in alcoholics, hepatitis patients, etc., with relative frequency. There is widely standing theory that NutraSweet and saccharin are stored in body tissues, possibly in the form of cellulite; and based on that reasonable theory, I would recommend all patients to stay away from those and similar type substances. Our goal is to maintain healthy detoxification pathways, maintain reasonable storages, and assimilate useful nutrients. As a result, we should have clearer thinking, more vitality and energy, and visibly better color and skin structure.

With excessive insults to the liver, it becomes less capable of performing vital functions such as helping to maintain the immunity, manufacture vital proteins and nutrients, and for assortment of various substances. It is obvious, for example, how dehydration alone might limit the capacity of the liver. This consideration alone can greatly benefit most patients, and therefore, a frequent and obvious recommendation is to get plenty of fresh water and herbal teas between mealtimes. Dilute your juices half and half with purified or distilled water to lessen the sugar content and improve water consumption.

Basic Understanding of Liver Detoxification Pathways

In general, there are three stages of liver substance detoxification. These pathways work together to break down substances and put them in a form that can be removed effectively from the body. These substances may include neurotransmitters, hormones, toxins, foodstuffs, metabolites, and even nutrients. These three stages are called phase 1, phase 2, and phase 3 detoxification pathways. Phase 1 includes the well-known cytochrome P450 and other initial enzyme pathways. Phase 2 involves conjugation, deconjugation, and other pathways necessary to make the substance more soluble in water. Phase 3 detoxification pathways are still poorly understood and are represented by an antiporter type system (an active portal in the cell wall) that directly and actively transports substances that

—

cannot be effectively processed out of the cells against a gradient. Phase 3 liver activities requires much more energy than the first two phases and is necessary for heavy metals and other toxins too challenging for the other phases.

Sometimes the P450 can be overstimulated, causing excessive demands on phase 2 pathways, releasing toxic byproducts into the liver to irritate the liver cells. The resulting depletion of phase 2 systems, such as glutathione peroxidase necessary for making toxins water soluble, allows irritation to occur on and in the liver cells, leading to potentially severe hepatitis. Hepatitis can be severe to even deadly depending on the reserves present before the overactivity and the amount of toxic exposure. This suggests why overly aggressive herbs and many pharmaceuticals can be so damaging to the liver.

Certain plants and pharmaceutical drugs can enhance phase 1 detoxification including the better-studied cytochrome P450. Many substances require this particular route of detoxification, and thus, this enzyme system may be overloaded or what is called up-regulated. This means more enzymes are activated and become available in this pathway, causing more rapid breakdown capabilities. Certain substances get a sort of preferential treatment, so there can be somewhat an unpredictable pattern of substance breakdown with certain substances getting broken down too rapidly and others not getting appropriately broken down. Many pharmaceutical medications affect the cytochrome P450 system, often resulting in up-regulation over a period of time. When time is not sufficient for the enzyme system to respond to the increased demands of the new substances requiring alterations, the substances remain in the bloodstream, potentially building to dangerous levels. Over a period of time, the enzyme system generally up-regulates (numbers and/or activity of enzymes increases), allowing more rapid breakdown capabilities. This is one of the major causes of tolerance to medications, even caffeine. As a result, over a period of time, this enzyme system can become relatively overactive, increasing demands in phase 2 detoxification pathways, leading to a buildup of free radicals and other harmful substances in the liver, again resulting in liver injury.

It is necessary to restore phase 2 pathways to protect the liver and allow for healing. Particularly sulfur-based herbs and nutrients play an important role here, as these tend to effectively scavenge free radicals. Important examples of these natural substances include MSM or methylsulfonylmethane, glutathione, amino acids such as cysteine and glutamine, the ever-present garlic, the impressive turmeric, and alpha-lipoic acid. I highly recommend all these substances in generous quantities especially when dealing with issues involving hepatitis of any form.

The phase 3 detoxification pathways are as yet poorly understood, more so than the other two pathways which still require much research and careful study. This pathway system requires significant energy as harmful substances are actively excreted from cells to be released outside the body. Hopefully one day, a full book can be completed with much insight to maximize and protect liver function.

Our Liver and Our Moods

Ideally, we begin to understand the vital role our liver plays to our overall health, and we choose foods and lifestyles that protect and support this organ. Living as pure a life as possible while recognizing that we will always be exposed to environmental as well as internal toxins is paramount to maintaining our vitality and enthusiasm. I say enthusiasm because it is well recognized, particularly in ancient medical systems, the significant role the liver has on storing and dispersing our emotions in the form of hormones, neurohormones, neurochemicals, and other substances not readily identified or understood. For example, it is well accepted that the relationship between hormones and our emotions, that a buildup of hormones results in feelings of aggression, depression, and changes in libido. When our liver is able to process these hormones completely with little obstacles, we are able to live a calmer more peaceful existence.

Anger and aggression in particular are emotions that can be stored in the liver when not appropriately resolved. These emotions, as well as others, can be repeatedly felt when certain toxic substances tagged to them are released again into the bloodstream, often in turn to be inadequately dealt with and repeatedly repressed. When the liver is allowed to clear the toxins that have built up, which may take some time, moods become more stable, outlooks improve, and further toxic emotions do not get presented to the liver for processing. In part, this is a biological basis for being careful what you allow your mind to dwell upon, which results in either an upward spiral or a downward spiral in how your life manifests. Don't choose to place demands on your liver that can better be avoided in the first place. This can explain why we sometimes get emotions of which we cannot identify the source of; the emotion is getting felt when the toxic substance it is tagged to is released spontaneously into the bloodstream. If we can process and excrete the toxic substance, the emotion tagged to it will resolve. As we reach a more pure existence, we have less spontaneous release of "repressed" emotions with resulting improved mental health.

It is important to forgive, for this reason, others as well as yourself. Guilt and blame are extremely toxic emotions for the liver to deal with.

Many spiritual people realize the importance of maintaining a more pure body as a means of being closer to God. When our liver in particular is running clean, we can be more receptive to our intuition as God's inner wisdom and guidance in our lives. In the Bible, our body is referred to as the living holy temple, and we are carefully instructed against defiling this temple. This by no means assumes healthy people are more spiritual and vice versa. It is just a suggestion that, as you strive for spiritual wisdom, it helps to keep your body as pure as possible for accurate reception. We

—

all come into this world with our own unique gifts and weaknesses, and it is important for each of us to find our own unique way. The goal is not of that of competition with each other for a seeming limited supply of spiritual gifts or health or other desirable materials, but for each of us to understand we are unique representatives of God, each with our own purpose and role to fill. We can succeed best as a group working together and encouraging each other. Allowing our liver to function efficiently and effectively allows us to maximize our own lives, thus benefiting those around us both directly and indirectly.

Interestingly, St. John's wort (*Hypericum perforatum*), an herb well publicized for its antidepressant effects in current literature, historically was regularly used for congested, turbid liver condition. Researchers have not been able to determine just how St. John's is effective and its mechanism of action. They continue to attempt to isolate constituents trying to find out the action relating to the nervous system. Could this herb be lifting depression simply by freeing up the liver? Respected alternative healers are considering this in light of St. John's wort's historical use as well as the improved liver function that is the result of this plant.

Maximizing Liver Function

After eliminating as many harmful exposures as possible, realizing you cannot be perfect, it is important to regularly take steps to help insure optimal liver function. These include simple things such as getting enough pure drinking water. As previously mentioned, water in almost all patients improves body functions as it supports the blood, the river of life.

Foods can also be incorporated into the diet that stimulate liver function, such as lemon water prior to a meal, salad greens with plenty of bitter greens early in the meal, and the consumption of olive oil to stimulate biliary flow.

Also, certain foods may be very helpful in providing nourishment to the liver with rapid cell growth and functions. In particular, dark green vegetables and carotene rich vegetables are beneficial. Artichokes contribute significantly to liver health as do beets.

Parasites should at least be considered as flukes and other pathogens can ascend into the liver by way of the portal duct or circulation, causing symptoms of gallbladder disease and nonspecific hepatitis. Although this possibility may be poorly accepted, it is because of this ignorance that we continue to harbor these organisms. At least open your eyes to this possibility, as this consideration adequately responded to can do much to improve your vitality. Good digestive and immune health likely benefits parasite issues.

In addition, it is not only necessary to know of and use herbs and supplements that improve liver function appropriately, it is necessary to both stimulate bile flow adequately and keep the bowels open. We do not want to stimulate a liver when the bowel is sluggish, as this would cause unnecessary stress and discomfort on the body. First, get the bowels moving regularly, daily, and then approach the liver. Also, be aware that you can use herbs, such as milk thistle acutely for poisonings and intoxications, with much benefit.

Lastly, when you are attempting to use herbs to cleanse to bloodstream, realize a major portion of this cleansing takes place in the liver. Be careful not to clean the bloodstream on a weakened liver, as you can significantly worsen liver function by overwhelming this organ with toxins trying to get excreted. If the liver is not functioning well, go very slow with your cleansing until the load is lessened and the liver has been built up. An example of this has occurred not too rarely where the herb chaparral, used in holistic cancer regimens, results in significant hepatitis from overwhelming the already weak liver in the cancer patient. Chaparral received a bad rap for "causing liver injury" while it was only doing its job. Cleanse the liver before you cleanse the blood, and you will get better, safer results.

Specific Herbs

Cellular protection
- Milk thistle seed
- Berries, bioflavonoids
- Schisandra root
- Licorice root
- Turmeric root

To improve liver cellular function and regeneration
- Milk thistle seed
- Dandelion plant
- Turmeric root (actually a rhizome)
- S. John's wort flowering tops, leaves

To improve biliary flow
- Barberry root
- Oregon grape root
- Dandelion plant
- Olive oil
- Yellow dock root

To aid in function and detoxification pathways
- St. Johns wort flowering tops, leaves
- Yellow dock root
- Oregon grape root
- Garlic bulb (sulfur)
- Milk thistle seed
- Dandelion, whole plant

To help bloodstream cleansing after above adequately functioning
- Red raspberry leaves-gentle
- Red clover blossoms and leaves
- Burdock root
- Echinacea root
- Nettle leaves dried or boiled
- Kelp whole plant
- Chaparral leaves—extremely powerful, use under supervision

To stimulate liver digestive activity
- Lemon (before meals in water)
- Bitter herbs (small teaspoon doses or so):
- Hyssop
- Yarrow
- Wormwood
- California poppy
- Coriander
- Curry

To improve appetite
- Barberry

(Appetite should improve anytime liver function is improved to some degree. Barberry is specific for this.)

Specific Supplements to Support Liver Function

Sulfur for detoxification pathways
- Glutathione
- Cysteine
- MSM

Cell protection:

- Alpha-lipoic acid
- Coenzyme Q 10
- Essential Fatty Acids (flax, borage, EPO, fresh nuts and seeds, avocado)
- Carrots (fresh juice, vitamin A)
- Vitamin C and E, selenium
- Sulfur

Cleansing

- Beet powder or juice
- Carrot juice

Obviously these lists are not complete but are here to give you some examples of the variety of approaches natural health can take.

Enema Therapy

The use of enemas can be very beneficial for liver function. The circulation of the colon goes directly to the liver, bringing the enema fluids directly to the liver unmodified by enzymes or hydrochloric acid. It is important that enema fluid be freshly prepared, brought to a boil and then allowed to cool, keeping the fluid relatively sterile. Be sure you tolerate the teas before you use them in the stronger enema form. Catnip is a particularly beneficial tea in enema form with its antispasmodic properties. You can be very generous in your use of catnip, red raspberry, and nettle-type teas, four teaspoons or so will give very beneficial and gentle results. But with respect to the liver, bitter herbs may be more effective in promoting the liver to dump its toxic load. Yarrow and hyssop in tea when formed as an enema can greatly alleviate liver toxicity with its associated symptoms of nausea, anorexia, and fatigue. It does not take a lot of these two though, for they can be quite powerful. Goldenseal is not recommended for this kind of use on patients with bowel complaints; goldenseal can be too irritating and eventually allergenic, the same is true with psyllium husks.

Organic coffee is also considered beneficial in enema form as, with the old saying "like attracts like," thus allowing the removal of toxins. Coffee, most importantly organically prepared coffee, can be very helpful as an enema for clearing the liver. I have read of a concern that coffee could bring toxins from a sluggish bowel into the liver with it, so again be sure the bowels are moving before you undertake enemas with the specific purpose of clearing the liver. Stay with catnip for a while before trying yarrow, which can elicit a remarkable healing response. Also, protect your kidneys from any toxic damage by adding some dandelion or marshmallow to your therapy. Use these herbs to not only in an effort to enhance bowel healing but also kidney health. Kidneys are involved in any cleansing process as toxins are released into the blood.

In general, I recommend combination teas for use as enemas. Catnip blends well with California poppy, which also is quite bitter. California poppy helps to relieve pain and spasms. Hops flowering tops is also very helpful for pain in this form. Hyssop also mixes with these nicely, and has significant cleansing and healing properties. Milk thistle would be at its' best. Use roughly a teaspoon of each. Don't make extremely complicated enema teas, this way if you get an undesirable action you get an idea which particular plant is involved. Always start with small amounts of familiar herbs. There is always a possibility of an allergic reaction.

Interestingly, I experienced almost complete, and at times *complete*, resolution of not only severe and chronic debilitating nausea but also severe allergy symptoms throughout my body with specific liver flushes by enema therapy. Fortunately, I rarely require any more antihistamines or nausea medications (also generally antihistamines.) I am grateful to

—

say my severe intractable nausea and allergies are both at a minimum if not asymptomatic. The symptoms may recur at a later date, but the teas are important therapies that should be utilized more frequently with care. Chronic headaches and cravings for harmful substances can be dramatically relieved with each treatment. I would only do one treatment a day for a week or so, then as needed. There is a tremendous role liver flush enemas may do in alleviating suffering. Much healing is possible with gentle herbal enemas. It is best to give the bowels a chance to heal and function before liver cleanses are undertaken. You do not want to further insult a bowel with liver toxins by being impatient with your healing. Also, start low and go slow. Ultimately, there is a strong possibility enemas will no longer be necessary as you heal. Enemas should only be taken with competent help.

Consider growing your own herbs. Harvest the flowering tops and other active parts of the plants and place in tea or carefully dry for future use.

Allergic symptoms may be a manifestation of liver toxicity, as the allergens cannot be processed and removed adequately from the overloaded organ. When the liver is running freely, these substances can be more effectively managed with less immune response throughout the body. I'm sure there is more to it than just liver dysfunction, but this organ is obviously a big player in allergy.

CHAPTER 7

Recognizing Food Intolerances and Allergies

Although there is much debate regarding the role of diet in certain disease like allergy, asthma and eczema, I cannot believe diet would not be playing a role in disease manifestation. There is much alternative literature, and ideas abound regarding the connection between food and health. One of the problems is defining food allergy. If you are only looking for skin sensitization with a histamine response, allergy has more limited definition. Common skin testing procedures available in most allergists' offices recognize this form of allergy.

I prefer to call other immune responses recognized in testing usually as IgG responses as food sensitivities. Sensitivities could be interrelated to food intolerances where you feel bad after you eat. Food intolerances though also constitute dietary limitations such as enzyme deficiencies and similar digestive weaknesses that allow food to ferment improperly rather than be absorbed. Obviously, infection such as food poisoning would be food intolerance. Digestive weaknesses beget sensitivities as well. Cow's milk for many individuals represents this type of complex intolerance. Most people lose the lactase enzyme necessary to digest milk sugars properly,

–
84

resulting in gastrointestinal symptoms such as bloating (fermentation). But we also have intolerance to milk because the improperly digested food is likely more sensitizing when chronically exposed in undigested form within the intestines. We do have antibodies within the intestines to block overload of antigenic substances (stimulate immune reactions), but especially over time and with repeated exposures or in especially deficient and delicate individuals, this protective antibody (IgA) is potentially overwhelmed. Consider this with the young who cannot tolerate cow's milk with their immature digestive linings. This could allow for much food sensitization and intolerance. I will try to refer to sensitivities as either allergic or immune-mediated and intolerance relating to the digestibility and its consequences. Food sensitivities do not necessarily equal food allergies.

Food sensitivities of this type are more difficult to recognize, and in Western medicine, there is much confusion to their validity. It is best to individually look at your own situation, keep a food diary, and note symptoms with times as well. After a period of time, you can find a clue to foods causing problems, try eliminating the foods as best as possible, and see for yourself if you or your child feels better. Some foods that are highly sensitizing, such as wheat and milk, are very highly pervasive in our cultural diet and must be more aggressively addressed. Trying to substitute wheat bread for rice bread is not an easy task. But interestingly, as the health connection is realized, the affected person often will eventually come around and realize the connection, taking more initiative in finding healthful foods. By observing dietary connections, mood disturbances, arthralgias (growing pains), insomnia, and other immune problems can be significantly alleviated. Autism as well has been increasingly associated with dietary and gastrointestinal problems and can be helped with nutrition. Other common findings with food sensitivities are hive reactions and swelling of tissues such as on the face, legs or abdomen. Along with nourishing foods and herbs to reduce this swelling, avoiding suspected

—

culprits may help to prevent reoccurrence. Of course, with hives and swelling, other possibilities may also be playing a role.

Various specific symptoms have been identified as possible effects of specific food intolerances. These symptoms vary relative to the person's innate constitution and tendencies. Areas of overuse and injury can often be predilection sites for specific immune complexes or reactivities. For example, knees often become painful when offending foods are eaten, especially when eaten regularly. Other medications and procedures may alleviate the pain, but the issue is never fully recognized or eliminated without the connection to the possible culprit(s). In contrast, some symptoms, by being related to constitutional tendencies, begin abruptly after the food is ingested and symptoms of reflux and heartburn manifest. We tend to eat the same foods so often we do not connect the association. Sometimes, the reaction is delayed, then it becomes more difficult to identify to culprit. Wheat may be okay for a day or two, and then three days later, you develop a painful joint. Often, food allergy/sensitivity symptoms occur symmetrically but not always to the same degree of intensity. One ankle may not be as painful as the other. This rule is obsolete in the case of an injury, which often becomes a predilection site for immune complexes floating around.

Another possible mechanism for food sensitization reactions is a cross recognition of the food particle with your own innate tissues. For example, heart muscle is similar, antigenically, to strep organisms. Therefore, with certain specific infections in this case, tissue damage occurs. A form of psoriasis is also the result of antigenic similarity confusion in the immunity. This same type of mechanism may be involved in food antigen similarities as well. Because this effect is not studied, we assume there is not a problem. But with increasing food sensitivity and unusual autoimmune syndromes, this theory should be recognized. I have tremendously benefited and have witnessed others benefits which may support this idea.

—

Good Habits Start Early

Again, teaching a child early about the importance of a healthful diet will go a long way in preserving his/her health and vitality. When we are young, we have more reserve; as we get older, we get less tolerant of poor habits.

Testing

As previously mentioned, skin testing is limited in its usefulness at detecting food sensitivity other than histamine-type responses that are only maybe half the problem with food intolerances. Some physicians who offer complementary approaches have blood tests that are more complete in determining IgG responses. These tests are somewhat expensive, roughly $300, but are worth the investment if you apply the results. It is helpful to specifically identify which foods you have developed immunity to. Then by avoiding the offending foods over a period of four months or so, your immunity to that food often will relax, allowing you to eat those foods again, albeit on a more limited method by rotating foods. It can be difficult to stay away from the offending foods, but by doing the best you can, you are decreasing hyperimmunity. Leaky bowel alone reasonably could have some IgG response, so you may be getting an indicator of the degree of leaky bowel you are dealing in addition to problem foods. Minimizing food sensitivities reasonably would improve bowel integrity. It is also important to maintain beneficial flora and exercise as possible to keep bowel functioning well.

The concept of food rotation is you must alternate the foods your body is exposed to. Leaky bowel is the result of yeast overgrowth, poor digestion, irritant foods, as well as food sensitivity itself. When the bowel lining is vulnerable, repeated exposures to same foods encourages sensitivity to develop. The more damaged the lining is, the worse the potential stimulus. The situation begets itself, as more immune reaction damages more lining. As the bowel is allowed to heal and become more intact by only allowing digested particles to cross, sensitivity diminishes, thus promoting further healing. By rotating foods, you are limiting the exposure to any one stimulus; if given sufficient time, the little immune response elicited relaxes, thus, never quite eliciting such as powerful and chronic immune reaction. Leaky bowel certainly can aggravate food sensitivities and vice versa. Not only must you care for the bowel and meet its nutrition needs while avoiding when possible insults such as antibiotics, but you should also limit food sensitization by rotating foods. We tend to eat the same foods daily; this habit should be modified to allow for rotation in the diet.

Earlier, when we did not preserve foods and transport them so readily, rotation was the rule. You ate what was available to the season. Fresh fruit in the summer, potatoes toward the fall and winter, etc., are examples of natural dietary rotation habits. Try to incorporate rotating the types of foods available to you and your children for optimum health and minimum sensitization.

Blood Testing

Blood testing, while informative, is obviously not the most available method of determining food sensitivities. Basically, you must draw out a test tube of blood, which is quite frightening for most children. The laboratory is able to determine quite a bit of allergy/immunity information with blood samples properly collected. There are a wide variety of assays and analysis that can be looked into. There are now many commercial laboratories that offer blood testing for sensitivities.

You especially may not want to subject the needle and collection procedure to very young children. In these cases, it is best to be very observant. Note colic, reflux, infection risk, rashes, and various "growing" pains. Although possibly there are legitimate growing pains, many currently identified as growing pains may indeed be food allergy symptoms. It is at least worth considering especially with any recurrent pains. You may try to test foods and substances by noninvasive testing, such as by muscle strength testing.

Strength Testing

Muscle strength testing is quite simple but takes experience and close observation. You might check your own strength testing first, put your dominant thumb and index finger together in a circle and find out how strong it is to pull the two fingers apart. Compare before and after exposures to chemicals, foods etc. To check someone else such as your child have your child close the thumb of his dominant hand to the index finger and find the force with your own hands of what it takes to open this ring, Checking strength responses to foods could be as simple as having the child flex his arm and determine the strength by noting how much resistance is present when you try to pull his arm down. Have the elbow on a steady and secure surface. Test the child's strength before and after the suspected food item is ingested. If you are highly worried about sensitivity, just have the child smell or hold the food in his other hand.

Pulse

Another possible approach is to check your child's pulse before and after ingestion of suspicious foods. Sensitivities can allow for increased heart rate, but this does not persist, so check early after the exposure.

Cravings

Cravings also not only may be the result of nutritional deficiencies but also the result of food sensitivities. Somehow through your body's methods of adjusting, it has learned to incorporate these immune complexes into processes in an effort to handle them. As the allergy continues, the processes developed to handle the insults become automatic, thus, causing cravings to continue to fuel the process. Cravings are very complex, but allergy or sensitivity may play a significant role. As you stop the offending foods, the cravings diminish with time. After a week or two, the cravings from sensitivity-related issues often are gone until sensitization reestablishes. After a month or so, you will not even desire the offending foods, although once in a while, you will surely miss them. They will not taste as good after sensitization is relieved.

Elimination Diets

It may be helpful to attempt to identify food sensitivities with elimination diets. Basically, you don't have the suspected foods available for at least a week if possible. Try to continue as balanced a diet as possible, substituting different foods with similar nutritional value. For example, to get a child away from wheat, such an absolutely notorious offender, especially in my home, offer foods prepared from corn and even rye. Rye is available as cakes, which is yeast-free as well; if you can adjust your children to these by placing tasty healthful garnishes as incentives, you can get the benefits of grain without wheat, less growing pains, and other reactions. Some families may have a predominance of corn or soy allergy, you must consider these as possibilities when evaluating your unique situation.

Dairy is another food that is best to eliminate from for at least sa couple months then maybe reintroduce in limited amounts and frequencies. Yoghurt may be more tolerated as it is pre-digested. You may be quite surprised at the symptoms that spontaneously resolve after you eliminate the offending foods. Later, when you do take in too much of the wrong foods for you, your body will more readily let you know. Thus, you become less likely to repeat yourself. Eventually, also your body will come to like the better foods in favor of the more harmful. Damaging food does not taste as good, or you only tolerate small amounts. It is very important to recognize the limitations to elimination of problem foods. Hazards such as parasites, deficiencies, yeast involvement, and food addiction cycles, all must be considered in effort to help adjust to changes in diet. Also, natural multivitamins are more important in this respect and possibly enzyme supplementation. Papaya might be considered as a regular part of the summer diet to aid digestion, for example.

When you apply the concepts of elimination planning, it is advisable to only eliminate one or two foods at a time. This allows you to fully appreciate the cause and effect cycle. Also, some sensitizers work together to augment your body's reactivity, for example, wheat with yeast, and coffee with sugar and dairy; in these situations obviously, it is necessary to omit multiple offenders. In the commercially available foods today, often multiple grains and food types are combined, complicating food sensitization. Another way to put it, you get wheat in almost every meal you eat every day. Rotation of foods is forgotten in our current culture. We make foods and even supplements so complex no one else can copy us; it allows our body to have chronic repeated exposure. Simplify.

Simplify your meals as well as your lives. Then it becomes more reasonable to rotate your foods and ultimately develop a healthy intestinal tract and few food sensitivities. Then occasionally, you can cheat on something you miss a lot and not suffer devastating or irritating consequences. Elimination diets take forethought and deliberant action as well as self-control. You must eliminate situations that cause you to fall and find appropriate substitutions you can get used to. Children nutrition can be challenging. It is difficult to protect your child from harmful foods without keeping them in the home all of the time. Peer pressure is significant, and children do not like to be seen as different. You might pack your child's lunch for the most part. When your child is young, it may be necessary to accept some improper food choices but kept to a minimum. Although ideally, the sooner you get a child into a healthful diet, the better for the child. Try to tell that to your seven-year-old who just doesn't understand.

Herbal Remedies for Food Sensitivities

In the cases where you or your child does get into foods that cause trouble, there are a few herbal therapies that may help. It is important to realize limitations to herbal remedies and to understand that avoiding the insult is much more effective and efficient than repairing the damage and limiting aftereffects. There are a variety of herbal remedies that can be helpful in alleviating reactions and minimizing damage. Some herbals can help support the body's reactions to stress, such as licorice root.

Licorice root, with its wonderful anti-inflammatory actions while supporting adrenal function (stress gland) should be considered in any severe or moderate allergic reaction. The sterol structures in licorice root are precursors and building blocks to adrenal products such as cortisol, thus in many ways, licorice can support a stressed adrenal. Licorice can be used in capsule, tea, and tincture forms. In some including children choose the glycerin tincture which is unfortunately not as easy to find. You might have to get the health food store to special order this or find a quality brand on line. Generally licorice root should not be used long term. Especially in significant doses there are cortisol-type effects from licorice root such as weight gain and high blood sugar. Possibly small doses of licorice root would benefit those under chronic stress, such as in chronic disease conditions. Larger doses should be reserved for more severe problems.

A much safer and more gentle approach would be to use the combination of astragalus and marshmallow. Astragalus, a traditional Chinese herb, is helpful for immune modulation. Marshmallow is an incredible immune modulator, and can be beneficial in all types of inflammatory reactions. Historically, marshmallow root has been regularly used for gangrene. The plant is helpful in many forms, and can be made into a glycerin tincture for use for children. Children usually prefer this to licorice; licorice has such a powerful taste. You also might try glycerin tinctures of lemon balm (Melissa) and/or catnip and fennel combinations widely available in many health food stores to help symptoms of swelling and bloating.

You also might benefit from the herbal teas you are now hopefully already incorporating in your diet rather than the many artificial beverages now commercially available. Find adequate refreshments that are nourishing and that meet you and your family's unique needs. Herbal teas that may help to calm an overactive immune system may include red raspberry leaf and nettle leaf tea. Catnip might be added to improve calming the child's nervous response to the offensive food. Children tend to like the taste of red raspberry leaf tea when fresh or properly prepared and stored. It is important to read the labels, as there is a lot of raspberry "flavored" tea, which may or may not contain raspberry. These plants could be grown in many climates.

Irritants

When you have allergies and sensitivities, it may help to completely avoid irritant foods and herbs. These certainly play a role in damaging intestinal lining aggravating food sensitivities. Peppers, strong spices, anti-inflammatory medications (OTC and Rx), and alcohol-based products can be harmful to the intestinal tract. In younger children the damage may be more severe. But even for adults, these foods and substances must be limited and respected. They potentially set up much allergy response. Glycerin tinctures may be more appropriate over the usually stronger alcohol tinctures.

Parasite infections also could be considered irritants. Depending on the number and the type of parasite intestinal permeability can by compromised. Do not assume like so many do that parasites are a normal part of life. Not if you are seeking optimum health. We have ignored the possibility of parasites for so long, the problem is potentially epidemic. Still quite undetected, only when certain obvious and loud cases get attention do we take notice at all. Unfortunately, this is to the detriment for our children and future generations. Parasites can potentially carry many organisms inside them thus enabling transfer more thoroughly and effectively. Improve your immune and digestive health, and parasites should not have such an easy place to stay.

Blood Type Considerations

Blood types and genetic patterns of ancestry can worsen sensitization or intolerance to certain foods. For example, the cruciferous family, including cabbage, broccoli, cauliflower, and many others, does better with certain genetic influences. Meat and dairy consumption is more tolerable and even beneficial to certain types. Sugars are better tolerated by those of European ancestry and Native Americans especially develop diabetes. Many do better on vegetarian type diets. Genetics play a significant role in the manifestations of symptoms.

Blood Type O

These people originally were hunters, traveling across the country. These people do best on animal protein and intense physical activity. These people have not adapted to dairy as well. They thrive on a high protein, low carbohydrate type diet. This allowed them to be lean and physical, necessary for hunting and gathering.

Blood Type A

This person is thought to be more delicate in the digestive tract. Type A developed later in history. They often farmed, and the blood type adapted from this lifestyle. More vegetarian in nature, over the course of time they adapted to more grains and vegetables. This type benefits from less and lighter meat consumption. Currently, nutritious and if possible organic grown foods do this type well. Seeds and legumes prepared properly allow for better protein assimilation.

Blood Type B

This person has a more robust digestion, and is more tolerant to stress as a result. He requires more balance in diet, physical and mental activity and can do well with dairy. In general he is allowed a more flexible diet.

Blood Type AB

This type developed later as the above types blended. Often with a sensitive digestive tract, the overall immune system is strong. These people do better with poultry and lean red meats. Properly prepared vegetables and wholesome grains are still important. For many they tolerate dairy in modest amounts.

—

CHAPTER 8

Toxic Exposures

There are great concerns regarding the environment and other health risks. A healthy environment usually means healthy individuals, especially children. When we take care of the world we are living in, the future generations will surely benefit. Reducing exposures to various pollutants most definitely improve the wellbeing and health of every person. Fresh air, peaceful surroundings, pure water, and fresh foods all are important, not one being more so than any other. They all work together for the benefit or detriment. Healthful attitudes and lifestyles also contribute significantly to the little ones vitality, and possibly contribute to healthy adulthoods. We must learn to protect and respect our environment more if not for us for our kids.

As I yell at my children for jumping on the furniture, I am reminded how difficult keeping a peaceful environment can be. It is not that we must be perfect, but we do our best to nurture surroundings for maximum spiritual, mental, and physical growth. Not that we should let our children run free rein, but they must have consistency as best as we can provide. Children benefit from knowing what to expect, from getting honest answers, and having predictable patterns in their life. So do adults. All this is reassuring and comforting. Growth involves discipline, when carried out and responded to appropriately and effectively. Life is not necessarily fair. It is interesting when I discipline one of my children, how they will later be calmer and more loving. I care enough in protecting them from things they should not do. We too have consequences for our actions. If you do not discipline your child appropriately, as God would, they do not think you care.

A healthy atmosphere, especially important for children, also must be maintained with awareness. Many of the television shows are inappropriate for young children even as background noise. Talk shows, news, and other dramas can be very alarming to the young minds that pick up so much more than you think. Children seem to have very large ears. The music also must be evaluated for the underlying messages it may bring to our children. We also should recognize the "spend—spend" mentality that causes our children to get more and more without real appreciation or value of what they already have. This can be a tough balancing act with all the peer and commercial pressures. Teaching your child early how to save, how to respect themselves and others, and how to control their thoughts toward good can start early. I tell my children for example to "speak and think life." Not only should you be an example of love toward your children in a healthy way, they should show that same example to others who may or may not have the guidance or consistency in their lives. We can set an example.

Children start out only thinking of themselves; this gradually should become a concern for others. For example, rather than focusing on whether someone loves me, focus on showing more love, in appropriate ways, to others. Start these lessons early and reinforce them by your own example.

There are other major considerations about the environment we surround ourselves in. Other than noise and mind pollution, we also must consider our water, air, food, and physical contacts. Many of the solvents, chemicals, and gases can be and often are harmful to both us and the

—

environment, especially over time. Evidence is everywhere if you look. Consider the scandal with the buttered popcorn industry; the workers sued the industry for millions because of exposure to the flavorings added to the popcorn.

Consider also the lifestyle, exposures, and eating patterns of ill versus well people. But keep in mind compassion; many have already started with limitations to their health, boundaries of what their body can handle. Others have robust constitutions that tolerate more. Indeed some individuals can actually tolerate quite a bit of insult without apparent harm. You must make your own decision about how far you will take this, but I will give you some examples of my gravest concerns:

- Aluminum
- Benzene
- Thallium
- Cadmium
- Mercury
- Carbon monoxide
- Lead
- Pesticides
- Chemical fertilizers
- Antibiotics
- Vaccines
- Chlorine
- Off-gassing from new furniture and newly painted rooms
- Synthetic foods (saccharine, etc.)

These various chemicals have a way of storing up in our body, possibly to manifest as disease later, especially with buildup on those at risk. In an effort to eliminate the potential problems ascribed to toxin buildup, we must learn first and foremost how to prevent the problem. We also must consider buildup from exposures that have already occurred and have not been dealt with effectively.

Teach your children *early* to avoid artificial substances as food and beverage in preference to wholesome foods and drinks. If we start with the youth, we may have a chance in getting some kind of control of diseases. Often diseases start their roots early, we just don't detect them until symptoms become increasingly clear and severe. It takes many years for these to manifest, only to take many quality years of life to reverse the condition if possible.

We can get exposure to many substances by inhalation and consumption but also do not forget the exposure to electrical currents and magnetic fields. It is true that certain magnetic fields may benefit health, although I personally do not use them; widespread exposure to large power lines should be avoided. Too much electrical magnetism can also come from the television, the computer, the various appliances we use. Be aware and minimize exposure.

Airplane radiation can be particularly innocuous but unmistakable effects occur with long-term exposure. Kelp can help with elimination of radiation exposure so, in present times, consider having ample supply of nourishing kelp. Also pure and even distilled water with lemon and salad bitters such as dandelions benefit cleansing out the residue from pollutants near airplanes and other gases. Juicing is also helpful in cleansing and many fine books are available on this. Carrot and celery juice can save lives. Beets are very powerful when juiced, and when combined with carrot juice is hard to beat for cleansing purposes. But don't do beets or even a lot of cleansing when pregnant as the pollutants and contaminants must travel the bloodstream to be eliminated.

Breathing exercises in areas with clean pure air can greatly benefit you, as can breathing in healing vapors of certain essential oils. We tend to breath too shallow. Breathe in, stop, and breathe in a little more. Hold and gently release. Feel your lungs expand with your hands on your lower ribs.

Pull the lower ribs outward gently. Appreciate whenever you are exposed to fresh pure air and don't waste any opportunity for the benefits of deep, relaxed, and controlled breathing technique.

So you can't escape the fumes all the time can you? Well, maybe those who live out on some beautiful estate with large trees and abundant flora with fresh water can. Purifying the air you live in is one option, and quality HEPA filters are helpful. Planting trees also can help add oxygen to our atmosphere, and any green plant has its value. HEPA filters must be chemical free and easily and readily changed. There are many to choose from, and generally, you do pay for quality. Be sure the filters are relatively easy to obtain.

Ionizers send out streams of negative charges, or ions, which are electrons to the atmosphere. These slightly charged (actually reduced) electrons find a target in the air, attach themselves, and then attach the particle more readily to any filter system as well as form dust. With these, you will notice more frequent filter changes are necessary as the air is effectively and safely cleaned. This method is relatively gentle. There are necklaces with ionizers attached that can be worn in places such as airports. Interestingly, there is a mountain climate in South America, a region of Ecuador, where people routinely live to be one hundred and more years of age; they have traced the possible reason as high negative ion levels in the atmosphere. The water was checked as well, but no difference was noted, only the ions in the air.

Ozonators are the opposite; they produce O3, which then detaches in the air to a particle, making O2. The positively charged oxygen (O) causes similar magnetic attraction, causing particles to effectively accumulate on filters or form dust. Ozone generators are wonderful sterilizers, quite effective, but powerful enough that you *should not breathe* the O3. Oxidation is damaging to delicate lung tissue as well as skin. It is good to use these in short bursts when necessary and then later in areas that require sterilization. I carried my ozone generator to work for urgent care;

people did not get ill from coming to a healthier environment. The central air filter would fill quickly and require more frequent replacement. Ozone is heavy so drops particulate to the ground. This was sufficient that the entire building took on a new freshness. Use ozone to sterilize vacated spaces. These units have specific instructions in their use and care is warranted to use them safely. Ozone generators are worth the investment in necessary conditions, just respect their power. Replace air conditioning filters as well as HEPA filters more often with these and ionizers.

HEPA filters are very useful. These can be quite effective in many areas, but get costly for larger or more heavily trafficked areas. They require regular and *frequent* filter replacement. The filters can add up in cost in heavily contaminated areas, a consideration that ozone generators can surmount, such as in sterilizing empty buildings. HEPAs and ionizers are very helpful in that there is no risk to breathing in any harmful ozone. Ozone is for places you can close off for a period of time and then let air out. Adequate air out time is essential, the ozone must drop out of the air before re-entry Especially with areas used in large gatherings, such as public schools, ionizers can be used regularly and ozonators ran for a short while at night, when the building is not occupied. These can be quite helpful and cost effective in keeping the germ and air pollution burden lower. The power of ozone is used in fire restoration. Ozone certainly could potentially damage lung and skin especially without adequate antioxidants in the diet (vitamin E, ginkgo, hawthorn berry, berries). Of course, cleaning as much as possible is still necessary in these high traffic and exposed areas; ozonators are not a replacement for adequate hygienic practices.

Water

Distilled water is quite helpful in healthful practices as this is the purest form. The distilled water should be placed in glass though, as the water is so "empty" that it will leach on any residue from plastic. So the best water is water purified or distilled by your own filters or distillers. But keeping bottled distilled water isn't a bad idea. Probably I would feel safest with purified drinking water rather than distilled water, but it probably is a toss up. The bottled distilled water is still good at pulling out the properties of the tea leaves and roots. Bottled water has benefits in convenience, but I recommend primarily drinking water that is purified with quality filters. Distilled water, which has no minerals in it, is preferred for making strong teas, as it extracts any substances it is exposed to. Distilled water can ultimately drain your body from nutrients if you are not cautious about putting good nutrients back. Water without minerals soaks up mineral deposits in a person but does not provide minerals back. You should take something loaded with organic minerals, such as kelp, alfalfa, dandelion, or nettle to replace and support mineral status. You can take these herbs at a different time from the distilled water if you are cleansing. If you just want a strong tea, take them together.

Not only educate yourself on water quality, but protect the environment's water contamination as you can. Clean up around your home, support wildlife, and do acts of kindness. Plant trees and shrubs that thrive in your environment although minimize plants that require much water in many areas in the U.S.

Watch out for the possible leaching of pollutants into ground water. Lead, arsenic, and others could certainly be damaging. Paint, paint thinners, auto oils all can be particularly a problem. Think about the world around you; get involved in your community.

Hair Analysis

Hair can be especially helpful in determining possible metal accumulation and risks. You should use hair from an area close to the scalp for the most current information. Hair does not necessarily accumulate toxins and metals but picks up whatever is in the blood. Hair is a long-term exposure picture. When hair has been died or similarly altered, obviously it may be more difficult to detect metal toxicity. Although I do not endorse any harsh chemicals that aren't absolutely necessary, especially on the head.

The skin picks up so much with the pores. Our skin is an important barrier but not impermeable. I don't even let my children draw on themselves or have tattoos, even the play kind, for fear of toxin exposure. It is up to you to protect our children, and ignorance about the toxicity and risks of metals and other contaminants is only now getting realized. Do not let ignorance prevent you from being responsible to your family and allowing your children the best chance at a vital future as God would plan it. Don't follow the pack but keep your path firm and grounded in knowledge and faith.

Hair is a good longer-term idea of circulatory toxins but not organ buildups, such as in the liver or even brain. It is very difficult to get accurate toxic loads but you can determine the risk by history usually.

Urinary Analysis

Urine is very easy and less disfiguring (for those who do not enjoy cutting off precious locks for toxicity tests). Urine suggests point in time circulatory toxic load; if you are detoxifying, you may actually have a high urine quantity. Low urine amounts of toxins alone do not tell you much but with history can be somewhat helpful. Blood levels result in urine levels but storage levels may be different, such as in the pituitary or liver.

DMPS Challenge

This is a way of causing your body to excrete more toxins into the circulation. After the kidneys filter the circulation, the urine can be collected and analyzed. This is a helpful way of determining body load. Experienced physicians should only perform this test as the detoxification reaction can be quite serious.

Assumptions

Another idea is to assume by your history the possibilities and gently but regularly complement your diet with bitter salads, juices, and other cleansing herbs. Occasionally drink distilled water in a mini-fast. With children though, you have the risk of hypoglycemia, they are so active and growing too. Encourage cleansing food; encourage cleansing red raspberry leaf tea. Give them fresh air and sunshine and green foods. Then assume you are protecting your children by being aware of possible exposures and preventing them as you are able. Encourage your children to eat leafy green lettuce, rich in color, as often as they will. Encourage them to chew slowly and to be relaxed.

Drink plenty of pure water and juices; grape juice is especially cleansing and nutritive. Grape juice can be sweet, so you might dilute it. Grape juice is usually the best tolerated by all types of people. Specific juices are better tolerated by certain constitutions maybe because of blood types and other genetic markers. Apple juice may be beneficial for some, but others may do better with orange juice. This is an individual thing. Apple juice might be best diluted in water for better effect. Learn what works best for you and your family members. But always drink plenty of pure water as well. Learn herbal tea blends your family enjoys.

Getting in the habit of drinking herbal teas is tradition in our home as the tea is almost always available. Kids have different needs. Our base tea is usually red raspberry leaf, easily grown here, and I add a variety of others depending on need. Red raspberry leaves are loaded with nutrients including iron. The vitamin C in red raspberry leaves helps our body assimilate this iron. Oh, there is so much we can learn from plants, especially about their healing and restorative properties when used appropriately and safely. Red raspberries and leaves can hurt no one. I have never heard of someone allergic to red raspberries. The plant seems easy enough to grow.

Some Specifics

Aluminum

This is everywhere. In bake-ware and cooking utensils, as well as antiperspirants and cosmetics, you almost cannot get away from it unless you understand the risk. Aluminum is also present in many baking products, for example, in baking powder, thus potentially threatening the industries involved by forcing them to find safer solutions. Awareness is the key. Don't use aluminum products. No aluminum foil. No commercial antiperspirant. No food made with aluminum cookery. Makes it seem hard, huh? Not really. At first, you may detoxify a bit; but after a week or two, you should be able to control perspiration with more healthful products. Crystals and natural products are constantly coming in the market. Seek aluminum-free products. A little certainly won't kill you and may not hurt you. Do not let aluminum become a problem through prevention. Aluminum is associated with at least Alzheimer's. Aluminum usually though is not looked for in disease. Read labels. Staying away from aluminum has helped our family stay healthy and hopefully will protect them from disease in later years.

Thallium, Benzenes, etc.

Chemicals from Styrofoam cups concern me greatly, especially when used by children. The hotter the drink, the more the ability to leach off any chemicals from the Styrofoam. I do not trust Styrofoam in my body. Styrofoam contains pseudo-estrogens that are carcinogenic. Many paper cups have plastic inner liners, and these can be good especially with cool drinks but also with warm beverages. Paper is the safest throw-away cup commercially available. There are probably many who would disagree and say there are also many chemicals in the bleached white cup. Anyway, these contaminants can accumulate and possibly contribute to diseases. I would especially recommend avoiding Styrofoam products with all the information available suggesting its contribution to disease. Styrofoam may be helpful as an outside surface with a completely lined cup, but even then you are dealing with a high cost to the environment your children must grow up in.

Glass is safe when not painted or treated with surface adherents. Plastic is safe when washed clean of chemicals and used for cooler food. Harder plastics can tolerate more heat still being safe. Styrofoam can handle very cool foods for a short while but, in general, should be avoided whenever possible. Styrofoam is also a mess to our environment. Be environment friendly as much as possible. Try to stay with paper cups for when you need to feed large groups. You could use quite thick paper but keep the chemicals out of it, or let the cups "air out" some. Off-gassing is the term used to describe the airing out of packaging and other products. A prime example would be to go into an unfinished furniture store where the wood has been treated with preservatives. Off-gassing of new products most often occurs early, upon opening the package, and other chemicals used to bleach paper or glue paper could be a problem.

Incidentally, newer packaging often contains Styrofoam, treated paper, and other thin plastics that are loaded with contaminants; do not breathe in the vapors or let your child inhale these fumes. Air everything out when you can. Frozen dinners obviously should not be a habit for the reasons stated above; the heat releases even more contaminants into the food. Once in a while is probably okay and even more than that for people with strong constitutions, but if you or your family is of delicate constitution, be aware of these exposure possibilities.

Mercury

I recommend total avoidance of amalgam fillings. Have them removed if at all possible. They leach (release slowly) mercury resulting in all kinds of intestinal problems at the least. Mercury (quicksilver) was used treat many kinds of disease and thought of as safe but has killed many instead. Now amalgams have somewhere around 50 percent mercury. In small chronic amounts, mercury could potentially wreak havoc, causing all kinds of poisoning. Mercury poisoning was associated with blackening of the skin, nausea, and vomiting. In heavy treatments, tissue would fall off. This debility was hard to manage in the early 1800s, but mercury should not be in use at all today. I am not alone in this concern over mercury still being in use in dental amalgams. Australia's governmental medical insurance pays for amalgam removals because of their understanding of the relationship of mercury to disease. I certainly have improved from places I have been health wise since the mercury fillings in my teeth were removed. I did have a mercury reaction though, as the blood had an increased load of mercury during the procedure. There are many testimonials. I have no doubt mercury can play a role in diseases today. Find a dentist who respects your wishes for mercury-free dental care.

—

Antibiotics

Antibiotics can be very useful but may be over-utilized rather than incorporating healthful practices of prevention. Antibiotics are fed to livestock for better outcome; antibiotics keep our children from perforating eardrums many times; antibiotics can be lifesaving but also misused. These should not be so freely utilized alone to care for a health problem. For example, using comfrey or plantain should prevent infection on a wound. Red raspberry leaves could help a lot of respiratory problems, as well as my favorite eucalyptus oil diluted as a rub and a steam inhalant.

Decreasing pollution would prevent and improve much disease. When people are in clean environments, their health improves. Consider how second hand smoke alone affects so many.

CHAPTER 9

Recognizing Your Child's Unique Weaknesses

Depending on the genetic predisposition as well as the environment, children develop with different strengths and weaknesses. Because understanding their individual weaknesses is important for the health and well being, I decided that a chapter on some of these possible weaknesses and how you might approach them should be considered. The expression of these weaknesses in the form of disease often takes time to manifest, so there is possible opportunity to prevent or minimize their expression. Attention deficit problems, irritable bowel, learning disorders, and skin disorders all are examples of problems that can be improved with healthful approaches. When children have these problems, it is important to continue necessary treatments and medications while you are nourishing the body. It is unfair and wrong to remove a medication that a child has become dependent on for the control of their symptoms. It is also a mistake to assume nothing can be done nutritionally and not attempt to meet the nutritional and environmental needs of the child, as these approaches offer long term benefits. Teaching children healthy living practices from an early age can potentially prevent further complications and chemical dependencies. This is not easy as children can be quite finicky. In general, the earlier you start incorporating beneficial practices in the child's life, the easier it is for them to adapt and develop good habits they can carry with them into adulthood. Stay flexible as you may get some resistance bringing in dietary changes. No matter what age we start, there is always room for improvement. We never stop learning.

It is very important that the close people in your child's life support healthy lifestyle habits. Friends, relatives, and schoolteachers have great influence over us, and they should recognize the benefit to your child, at least over a period of time. We are all setting examples to others. Remember, you are the one ultimately responsible for your child's growth and education not accessory people in your life. Take this responsibility with honor and privilege, remember all good things come from God and children most certainly are gifts. Also, take the initiative to find out what your child does well with and expand this understanding. Remember what works with one child may not work with another although children of the same genetics tend to have many of the same nutritional considerations. We are all on a continual learning curve, do the best you can and forgive yourself and others for things of the past. All we can do is the best we can at the time.

Gastrointestinal deficiencies

Our digestion is of vital importance in maintaining health by providing nourishment and waste removal. This is likely the first system that should be addressed when we are dealing with any health issues. Is the child constipated, meaning inadequate removal of waste products allowing for toxins to accumulate both in the bowel and blood. Ideally, a child should have at least two soft-formed stools daily, and generally the number of meals should roughly equate with the number of bowel movements. This is contrary to popular misconceptions that we do not necessarily need to have daily bowel movements. Over a period of time, constipation does cause disease, consider the problems with irritable bowel syndrome, diverticulitis, and colon cancer—these are all conditions that involve constipation. all well recognized to occur as a result of constipation. As our diets become more refined and concentrated, we slow bowel function. The muscles get weak, and thickened mucous, similar to sludge, builds up throughout the intestines especially the colon. Malnutrition and autointoxication which is the absorption of wastes into the blood both occur. Autointoxication refers to various byproducts of organisms as well as food metabolites and other substances getting absorbed into the bloodstream in toxic amounts. This can result in a variety of complaints from nausea, to headaches, to various aches and pains as these toxic products accumulate. The liver is over stimulated in attempt to clear the toxic materials. Overall, this excessive activity requires energy and results in nutritional deficiencies and fatigue.

Be sure your children are getting the best quality food you can obtain. Avoid preservatives, colors, and other chemical additives whenever possible. Be sure the oils your child ingests are of the best possible quality to support healthy cells. Minimize or even avoid artificially saturated oils. These are in a form that is very damaging to tissues, especially those involved in circulation where these damaging oils have much exposure. Circulation is important for all tissues. Cholesterol is a marker for circulatory health. Consider the problems with heart disease in younger and younger victims. Avoid margarine and rancid oils. Although butter is considered harmful to many, butter is actually *much* safer than margarine. Butter supports colon health. Our liver is necessary for the production as well as elimination of cholesterol, keeping the liver functioning optimally and clear will do much to improve cholesterol. Liver health greatly influences how we feel. A way to check liver health is with blood work. Measuring liver enzymes in blood work is of limited value in estimating liver health. Normal liver enzymes on blood work only suggest the liver is doing well. The liver can be very congested and poorly functioning with normal liver enzyme levels. These levels only suggest what is spilling out into the blood from damaged cells. Many factors can alter these levels; for example, what if the enzymes are so deficient there is little to spill? What if the cells are fat full of waste materials but not spilling at all? Symptoms and energy levels often can give you an idea of liver function. Back to butter. Beneficial bacteria in the gut support the liver. Butter has a component in it, butyric acid or butyrate, which actually has been found to be protective against colon cancer, presumably by supporting beneficial bacteria.

Polyunsaturated oils are nutritious. Olive oil is a healthful cooking oil. For baking canola oil is a good choice. When you cook or bake, be sure to use fresh oils; these tend to be unstable in heat and go rancid quickly. Taste the oil. The oil should taste fresh, smell fresh, and not have a "bite" to it. Use polyunsaturated oils whenever possible. Encourage your children to eat fresh green salads with polyunsaturated fresh oils on a regular basis. Make them eat a bite or two of avocado, unless you have determined they are allergic, very rare for children, regularly to provide them with high quality oil. Also, supplement your children with flaxseed oil. Because there is so much poor quality, damaging oils, you must make meeting nutritional needs of beneficial oils a priority. Certain fats cannot be synthesized in the body, the essential fatty acids. It is absolutely necessary to provide an adequate source of these to protect childhood development. These oils are necessary for the function and growth of every cell in our body, particularly those in the nervous system, circulatory system, and immune system. The nervous system depends on relatively large amounts of fatty acids for healthy function. Also, tissues that undergo rapid turnover, replacing themselves in a short time will be quickly affected by nutritional deficiencies such as inadequate intake of polyunsaturated and essential fatty acids. Our gastrointestinal lining cells very rapidly turnover, causing the gastrointestinal system to be quite vulnerable to malnutrition. We will see the early effects of malnutrition in the skin and hair as well. The skin may not heal well, be pale, be dry. Conditions such as eczema may get worse. In these cases, be sure to supplement beneficial oils. Prolonged malnutrition affects tissues that turn over more slowly such as the nervous tissues. These effects are later and take longer to improve. Learning disabilities and attention deficits benefit from good nutrition, but it does take longer to appreciate the benefits. Essential and polyunsaturated oils play a large role in nervous system development. Other nutrients should also be considered in these cases, but fatty acids are an important factor in the rise in problems with nervous system development.

To maximize digestion and nutrition, it is not only important to choose healthful foods but also combine them for the best absorption and assimilation possible. Absorption refers to the process of breaking down nutrients and bringing the nutrients into the bloodstream to provide for the various cells of the body. Assimilation is different; this refers to the process of various cells throughout the body incorporating the nutrients into tissues. For example, calcium carbonate, a pet peeve of mine, is often used to supplement foods with calcium. You will see the labels touting a good source of calcium. The labels are referring to a large amount of calcium added into the "food" though not necessarily a good source. Calcium carbonate is the forerunner of an absorbable but not assimilable substance. This particular calcium is not organic, not incorporated in plant material. Because of this, the calcium cannot be incorporated appropriately in cell structures, leading to the accumulation of this substance in deposits throughout the body. Isn't it interesting that with all the calcium supplementation and cow's milk ingestion, we have so much neurological deficits and osteoporosis? Why is calcium deposited in our arterial walls and joints but we still have brittle bones? On the other hand, patients who take calcium in the form of leafy green vegetables, celery, carrots, and other "organic" substances do not experience these problems. Cow's milk is of a different process though; this milk, although possibly considered organic, is poorly assimilable. This is due in part to food intolerance, to high protein content, and high phosphate content of cow's milk. In children, this is even more important because of their active growth.

With dietary approaches, basically simplify. Processed foods with a large variety of ingredients tend to be poorly digestible and mucous forming. Mucous forming refers to a process of thickening of mucous that should normally be watery. This thick mucous accumulates and passes through the body slowly, giving harmful bacteria a foothold. Watery mucous tends to wash out harmful bacteria and waste products readily. As the late Dr. Christopher put it, flour and water make "glue." This glue can be detrimental to the development of a child as well as the health of anybody. It is necessary to get adequate fluid intake in the form of pure water, but it is best to drink more between meals rather than with meals. Drinking too much fluid with meals dilutes salivary enzymes, which are very helpful for thorough digestion. Whatever foods are not digested pass on to the colon where they ferment. This is one of the reasons it is so necessary to address this. On the other hand, dehydration because of inadequate fluid intake contributes to constipation. Both processes aggravate autointoxication. There are various important "friendly flora," necessary for the breakdown of certain metabolites as well as the production of certain vitamins, so bacteria is necessary; it is a matter of how much and the types inhabiting the colon.

Sugars promote yeast, normal in small quantities, which can become pathogenic and invasive when allowed to proliferate excessively. Because of our children's excessive use of sugars, not only is it increasingly common to have yeast overgrowth situations but also important minerals required in the metabolism of sugars become depleted. This is the mechanism. White sugar is cane sugar with the minerals removed. These minerals constitute the blackstrap molasses available in health food stores. Our body requires these minerals to utilize the energy of the sugar. When we ingest white sugar, we must draw on other mineral reserves for effective metabolism. For example, you need calcium to contract a muscle. When we ingest or feed our children white sugar, we ultimately deplete body reserves of minerals, especially from the nervous system. Ultimately, sugar overuse results in nervousness. I understand it is difficult to get away from white sugar, do the best you can. With some children, this is easier than others. If your children do get white sugar, be conscientious in restoring the minerals. Consider supplementing your child with a lot of leafy green vegetables as well as a teaspoon or so of blackstrap molasses when necessary. Do not necessarily wait until you have outright symptoms of nervous deficiency to supplement (for example nervousness.) Children need balance, consistency, and ample reserves to support their rapid growth and from environmental stresses.

Yeast also causes its own havoc; it promotes hypoglycemia and irritability as a result. When too abundant, it is a chronic stress to the immune system in particular. Minimizing sugar usage may alleviate yeast overgrowth, although sometimes you cannot get the sugar usage down significantly until the yeast overgrowth is addressed. Yeast overgrowth understandably can lead to hypoglycemia that can result in uncomfortable sugar cravings. If you rid the body of the excessive yeast burden, often sugar cravings will remarkably improve.

Excess sugar can stress the adrenal glands, the organs responsible for stress management. With nutrient depletion and recurrent hypoglycemia, the adrenal glands become fatigued over a period of time, contributing further to disease. The excessive yeast burden also contributes to adrenal overload. The adrenal glands modulate immune function among other stress responses, which in turn poorly functions. All this contributes further to poor health. In addition, look at the harm these sugars do to our children's teeth. Teeth can be very expensive. Don't just brush them more although do this too, but minimize sugars. Dilute fruit juices half and half with water and avoid sodas as much as you possibly can. These good habits will go a long way in protecting your child's health. Herbal teas, lightly sweetened, also contain valuable minerals. Red raspberry leaf tea is our favorite, loaded with calcium, iron, and other valuable minerals. A great mineral-rich herbal tea blend my children love is a mixture of red raspberry leaf, nettle leaf, and hawthorn berry flower tea. I mix a few bags of each or a couple teaspoons of each in a pot of boiling pure water for an excellent nutritional beverage. I do use sugar modestly because it encourages my children to drink the tea abundantly, but I compensate with other minerals for any sugar I use. It is important to stress the usefulness and value of honey as a sweetener. Honey is loaded with minerals and beneficial enzymes, is anti-infection, and helps restore energy levels. An excellent source of minerals other than blackstrap molasses is kelp and dulse (seaweeds), available in health food stores. I put a few drops into their diluted juice to further improve their mineral balance. Also, there are quality mineral supplements widely available. Whole food concentrates and natural vitamins are also available although more costly. These supplements can be especially helpful for finicky children.

Ideally, don't introduce your children to sugar at an early age. Rather than sweet bananas, start babies with bland foods and vegetables. This may go a long way in teaching our children's taste buds healthier habits. Once our children get used to sugar, the taste buds have much difficulty reestablishing healthful preferences. You can also see this with salt; as most know, the more experienced cook tends to use too much salt. Our taste buds can be quite tricky and demanding. Especially with children and all of their exposure to concentrated sweets. Do not rely on misinformed taste buds as to what foods are good for you. We do have cravings to foods we need, but usually, the cravings are a result of hypoglycemia, food allergy, and habit. It is interesting to watch cravings disappear when yeast are eradicated effectively and when food sensitivities are eliminated for a week or so.

Hypoglycemia and Hyperglycemia

Sugar is the major energy currency in the body, especially necessary to feed the brain, which relies on available blood sugar as its primary and almost sole energy source. Other tissues, such as muscle tissue and liver tissue, can also utilize fats and ketones derived from fat. This is why sugar balance is so critical to health. Poor food choices play a major role in the development of abnormal blood sugar levels. The pancreas becomes too reactive to sugar loads, causing symptoms of hypoglycemia. When we eat simple sugars, they are quickly absorbed into the bloodstream, raising blood levels of glucose rapidly.

When we ingest a significant amount of simple sugar in the form of white sugar or white bread, for example, it is the responsibility of our pancreas to release adequate insulin to utilize the sugar entering the bloodstream. Cell membranes have insulin receptors that allow the insulin to bind to the cell and stimulate the uptake of sugar into the cell, therefore, removing the sugar from the blood. It is especially important for muscle and fat tissue to have adequate receptor responsiveness to bind the insulin and allow for the uptake of sugar for use or storage. The more responsive pancreas that rapidly secretes insulin keeps the blood sugar more stable by minimizing the rise in the blood sugar level. As the insulin enters the bloodstream, it causes the insulin-binding receptors to react, eventually losing their sensitivity to the insulin, causing insulin resistance. As we age, the insulin resistance gets more profound, causing obesity first as insulin is over-utilized and later adult onset diabetes or the "metabolic syndrome." This is a "new" syndrome that has insulin receptor resistance as its most obvious characteristic.

It becomes very important therefore, to start our children on a healthy diet from early on, as diabetes and the metabolic syndrome, both a result of insulin resistance, are epidemics, especially in our own country. Repeatedly overloading the system with refined sugars is the primary cause for insulin-resistant diabetes (type 2 adult onset). It is important to distinguish the difference between insulin-resistant type 2 diabetes (adult onset,) and type 1 diabetes (juvenile onset.) Type 1 diabetes is more related to pancreatic failure, possibly from autoimmune reactions to the pancreatic cells, the beta cells of the islets of Langerhans. These are the cells responsible for insulin secretion. As these cells are destroyed, insulin responses become increasingly limited and eventually fail in most cases. Sugar overdoses aggravate non-insulin resistant diabetes (type 1 juvenile,) before the pancreatic failure is complete by placing excessive demands on the failing organ. After the pancreas has failed in producing insulin, the sugar must be compensated for with the administration of insulin by injection, insulin cannot be taken by mouth. Why we form these antibodies (autoimmunity) is still subject to speculation. I would recommend cleansing and antiparasitic treatments. Also I would recommend pancreatic supportive herbs such as mullein, cedar berries, and uva ursi taken over a long period of time in moderate doses to attempt to restore pancreatic function by supporting the pancreas nutritionally. There are success stories of people overcoming diabetes, but this takes diligence. Also, follow the principles outlined below for insulin resistance.

Of course, some people are at more risk for developing diabetes than others based on their hereditary risks. It is well known that Hispanics and American Indians now have an increased risk of diabetes. As people move to a more refined diet, their risk increases. For example, Japan now has an increased risk for diabetes types of problems.

Insulin resistance can be suspected when a patient is overweight. Also, people can get a darkening of the skin that is highly suggestive of insulin resistance. The way to cure this problem is to lose weight and change your diet. Be sure to incorporate valuable essential fatty acids in your diet, as I see a correlation between these and cell membrane health and insulin receptor response. In fact, I believe essential fatty acids are a major missing link to the whole metabolic syndrome, a process poorly understood on a nutritional basis. Obviously, adequate vitamins, minerals, and balanced protein are also important for healthy cellular functions. Exercise is especially important for people suffering with metabolic problems, and even daily walking for a half hour can benefit profoundly when done consistently.

Our liver is responsible for storing readily available sugar for rapid breakdown should our diet not supply enough sugar on its own. When we are fasting or under chronic stress, our liver receives messages to release this sugar into the blood. This supply eventually will be depleted though and then we synthesize sugars from proteins. At a later time, we restore this reserve when we eat a meal.

Hypoglycemia occurs when the blood sugar falls too low, causing symptoms of weakness, nausea, lightheadedness, agitation, hunger, and even coma in severe cases. This can occur when we do not eat enough or digest foods well. This type of hypoglycemia may occur with fasting for extended lengths of time or performing excessive activity, allowing for the depletion of liver sugar reserves. This is not the common cause for the hypoglycemia of the children today. Hypoglycemia usually occurs when there is too much insulin. This can happen with over-medication as well as over-stimulation by the pancreas by excessive sweets.

Our children are usually getting hypoglycemia from eating sugary foods rapidly and repeatedly. As our body adjusts to the expected sugar intake, our pancreas automatically secretes insulin, sometimes even prior to actually eating the sugary food. Therefore, we may react to the food in anticipation of the food, such as people who get addicted to donuts in the morning. We see or expect or smell the food, we secrete insulin; as a result, we become hypoglycemic, causing us to demand the food. Also, when we eat the sugary food, our body learns to quickly neutralize the threat of a high blood sugar, causing the body to overreact, secreting relatively too much insulin because of the excessive stimulus, causing the sugar to plummet to levels lower than normal. Then we get cranky and weak and

—

eat more sugar to overcome the symptoms, setting up the cycle again. To alleviate these problems, we need to frequently eat smaller nutritious meals while replacing necessary nutrients with super foods such as spirulina and blackstrap molasses, honey, and oats.

Hypoglycemia may result from yeast overgrowth as yeast organisms thrive on sugar. Not only do sugars promote the growth of pathogenic yeasts, yeasts in turn cause more cravings for sugars. In these instances, it is best to promote a yeast-free diet while taking medications, herbal or pharmaceutical, to eradicate overgrowth of yeasts. Patients suspected to carry yeasts overgrowth tend to have sugar cravings, poor attention and memory skills, fatigue, and severe immunological imbalances such as allergies, autoimmunities, and deficiencies. When you are considering the role yeasts may play in your own unique circumstances, also consider parasites. Treat these infections. Do this slowly and carefully, allowing the body to completely restore and rebalance itself. As always, support good nutrition and immunity to minimize the risks of these infections.

Mood Disturbances

Children can be born or develop deficiencies in their nervous system, manifesting as mood disturbances. This may include attention deficit, depression, irritability, insomnia, and others. It is especially important for the nervous system so rapidly growing to have its nutritional needs met. Getting quality fatty acids, including the essential fatty acids, is quite important as is getting balanced quality protein and vitamins and minerals. The best source for these substances is from wholesome foods. Teach and practice healthy eating habits early.

Nervines, herbs that support nervous tissue, may play a special role in supporting nerve development and function by providing vital nutrients. Nutrient deficiencies indeed can be generational, passed down in the family for generations by way of genetics. Nervines serve to support and help correct imbalances. Nervines also can help support nervous tissue chronically neglected or overlooked that needs regeneration. That covers many of us. Use herbs such as skullcap, catnip, blue vervain, blue cohosh, and passion flower on a low dose and continuous basis for best results. For acute problems with nervous exhaustion, you may use catnip or Melissa in larger doses. The glycerin tincture works effectively for acute treatment, although teas can be given regularly that support the nervous system. My favorite blend, red raspberry and nettle leaf, in this case with catnip, can be a quite soothing tea for children, as well as adults, especially when prepared with honey.

The nervous system depends on a healthy myelin sheath around many nerves to smooth and control function efficiently. This particular membrane has a high quantity of essential fatty acids, although these are necessary for all cell membranes, not just nervous tissue. Quality dietary fish may play a helpful role in supporting nervous system development. Fish is well known to contain beneficial fatty acids that are necessary for nervous system maintenance. These particular fatty acids, eicosoepiandosterone (EPA) and docasohexanoic acid (DHA) either must be supplied by the diet or manufactured in the liver from omega 3 essential fatty acids. A great source of omega 3 precursors for DHA and EPA is flaxseed oil. If the child or patient has liver function deficiency, which is usually reserved for more elderly or very toxic children, then you might consider supplementing with DHA and EPA directly from a fish oil source. Evening primrose oil is considered to be very nutritive to the myelin, and has been helpful in many patients suffering from multiple sclerosis, a myelin inflammatory disorder. Remember to refrigerate these valuable oils to help preserve them and discourage rancidity. These oils should smell fresh. Also, olive oil itself is valuable to support nervous tissue. Remember your oils.

Getting quality vitamins and minerals also is very important to support nervous system development and function. As previously mentioned, you might consider supplementation with blackstrap molasses to provide quality calcium and magnesium, among other important minerals. Herbal teas also contain valuable minerals and trace minerals, for example nettle leaf and red raspberry leaf tea. Honey can be helpful here. Dark leafy green vegetables and carotene rich (orange) vegetables are also particularly useful in feeding the nervous tissue. The chlorophyll in dark leafy green vegetables, herbs, and foods can be quite restorative to nervous tissue as well, in mechanisms not totally understood. Chlorophyll rich foods are important detoxifiers, as well as oxygenating to help allow tissues to repair effectively and efficiently.

A Note about Autism

Autism affects many. These individuals have difficulty in communication, both within themselves and to others. Good prenatal and postnatal nutrition are important but when you are working with an affected person consider the colon health. Autism symptoms may improve with attention to colon health using probiotics. This may be a significant help to some parents, as they try to get their children to communicate more effectively. Work on intestinal flora health; avoid antibiotics whenever possible, choosing more benign treatments such as garlic in honey in frequent doses. Use probiotic supplements that come from a reputable distributor. Your child may not require these for an extended period of time, just long enough to recolonize his intestinal and body microflora in more protective ratios. Avoid dairy. Again, eradicate yeasts and parasites. Encourage your carrot and celery juice to improve mineral and vitamin status in an effective way. Even just a sip daily if you can. Do this over a period of time, not a week. Give the child time to adjust to the bodily changes with plenty of nutritious foods and beverages. Never give up on helping your child be able to communicate effectively, this is so important. When a child's nervous system is nourished, he can not only relate more effectively to his environment but also to his own internal communication of understanding what he is feeling and what he needs.

Poisonings

Another very important consideration with children with mood disturbances such as depression is toxic exposures. This may be heavy metals, chemical contaminants, or food additives and colorings that your child may be sensitive too. All of these problems can coexist. There are two effective ways to determine heavy metal poisoning, hair and urine analysis. Blood levels may not adequately qualify the extent of the poisoning because the metals do not remain in the blood but are stored in areas such as the liver, the brain, and other organs. Hair may be an effective way to get a crude assessment of heavy metal and mineral overdoses; this test is available from knowledgeable natural health care providers and certain health food stores. The test does not require a prescription. You just send a sample of new hair growth, not the ends of long tresses but the more time-accurate newly grown hair close to the scalp. The test may be worth the investment and loss of hair. In return, you receive a detailed report of heavy metal exposure as well as mineral status. Then you can be better equipped to identify the source of the problem. Along these lines, do not let you dentist use amalgam fillings in your child's teeth. Mercury, a significant percentage (to 50 percent) of amalgam fillings, has no business in your mouth. This metal destroys enzyme activity, accumulates in important areas such as brain tissue, and causes much morbidity that may not be associated with its use. If you apply one suggestion I give, at least make it this one. Mercury in amalgam fillings may contribute to chronic health problems later in life, as the metal leaches out into the body. If you already have these fillings, get them out if you can. No more, the more mercury the worse off you will be. Find a qualified dentist willing to help you and make the investment to get these fillings out in trade for porcelain or composite restorations. Certain herbs can help you detoxify mercury, especially chlorophyll rich herbs such as kelp. Red clover may also help. There are also pharmaceutical medications used to remove stores of mercury; these require the prescription and supervision of a qualified physician. Do not remove all the harmful fillings at one time, but do this in a sequential manner to limit toxicity from the mercury released during the procedure. Do not swallow your secretions and water the dentist uses to rinse your mouth; spit all this out as best you can.

Another very common pollutant in our body is aluminum. Although there is a significant amount of literature available denouncing the use of aluminum in cookware and soda cans, the industry has been present for so long little is done about the concern. This is similar to mercury; with all of our scientific knowledge, we forget common sense. Because these metals only cause damage over an extended period of time, unless in extreme quantities, we assume there is no damage. Also, different people have different susceptibilities. Unfortunately, later we develop all the mysterious disease's syndromes that we cannot understand how it developed. We ask, why me? Haven't changed anything in the diet, can't be the soda cans, been doing that for so long. Where did this cancer come from? Rather than assuming the food industry is at all concerned for your health and blindly trusting that anything called food is okay, educate yourself and take responsibility. This is especially important as our environment continues to become more toxic and foods more processed. Again, consider a hair analysis to get an idea of the pollutants you may be dealing with; do this earlier rather than later to minimize unnecessary symptoms and disease.

Especially look around the environment and at the food labels. Food additives used to preserve or enhance the flavor of foods are often implicated in nervous disorders, especially symptoms of hyperactivity and attention deficiency. At times it is necessary to medicate a sufferer with attention or behavioral approaches, but include a healthier diet which does additional benefits. With these children in particular, it may be a valuable habit to avoid processed foods altogether. Pharmaceuticals only manage symptoms, not underlying causes, and therefore allow the causes to continue. It can be very unfair to expect a child with sensitivity to food additives to control his behavior by counselling alone, but pharmaceutical drugs alone are not the answer either. Consider using nervine herbs to nourish the nervous system and promote healing while doing your best to avoid harmful substances.

Is the air fresh, is the energy positive in the environment. These are other environmental factors to consider. Open your windows when you can. Have some living houseplants to absorb pollutants and provide fresh oxygen. Consider investing in air filtering systems, there are so many types to choose from available. Also, minimize your child's exposure to electromagnetic fields, another possible source of toxicity. Watch out especially for large power lines, move away from these. Keep electrical appliances away from the bed, especially the head of the bed. Have your children sit back and away from the TV, stand back from the microwave, and other appliances. Don't use the alarm clocks that have the red led lights unless you keep them several feet from the bed. Avoid electrical wires under the bed as well. Also minimize use of electric blankets; use fine wool or other natural fiber blankets instead.

Another consideration to children's mental health is to avoid manmade fibers in clothes in favor of natural fibers, organic if possible. Synthetic fibers have electrical charge and also do not allow the skin to breathe. Natural fibers are considered to be of higher vibration, this being conducive to health. Silk, cotton, hemp, linen, and wool all have very high vibrations. Our skin is considered our third lung by most natural healers both in the past and in the present. Even though polyester nightgowns are

—

soft, they do not promote health. Choose cotton instead. Lower vibrational energy is associated with confusion, deception, and death. This relates to our clothes as well as our foods and lifestyles.

Allergies and Asthma

Children suffering from these complaints can be very limited in their performance and learning ability, being distracted by the illness as well as the medication side effects. Children with allergies and asthma are also likely suboptimal nutritionally due to the factors that may be giving rise to the allergic symptoms. These children do not sleep well and often deal with significant fatigue from both this lack of adequate sleep but also from the excessive waste of energy their body is undergoing from this unnecessary hyperactive immune response. In addition, children with asthma have increased work in breathing, which over time results in additional fatigue as well as possible suboptimal oxygenation. While these children's issues are being addressed, it is particularly important to allow them adequate rest.

Children can develop recurrent infections when their immune system is not functioning optimally. It is important to address the underlying imbalances. Healthy intestinal microflora balance and promote optimum nutrition. In children, recurrent infections can be a symptom of underlying toxicity from an accumulation of mucus waste products. Again, avoid refined sugar, flour, and dairy to improve the mucus function and make the mucus more watery and therefore slippery. Thick mucus is asking for infection. Work on a cleansing routine to help prevent infection.

Two areas may be worth pointing out. If the recurrent infections involve the urinary tract, it is helpful to use soothing herbs with a affinity for the urinary tract, such as marshmallow root. This herb is widely available and easy to grow, useful both in a tea form as well as a glycerin tincture. It is probably better to avoid alcohol tinctures when possible, especially in children, for many cannot tolerate alcohol even in these small quantities. Usually though, it takes less alcohol tincture to get the results desired, so if you must use alcohol tinctures, just drop them in hot tea, stir, and give a little time to allow the alcohol to evaporate. Gravel root and hydrangea root also are extremely valuable urinary tract remedies with cleansing and soothing properties. Uva ursi has some antibiotic action and may be used as well, but I would recommend combining it with some of the abovementioned herbs for their more soothing properties. Especially avoid carbonated beverages; these are extremely toxic to the delicate urinary tract. I would attribute a large percentage of urinary tract problems to the use of these drinks, which should be avoided. Cranberry juice has a reliable use as an adjuvant in the treatment of urinary tract infections; the juice limits the ability of bacteria to attach to the urinary tract lining. Cranberry juice is alkalinizing, another process that inhibits the growth of bacteria. Drink plenty of herbal teas as well as pure water to promote cleansing of the urinary tract by maintaining generous hydration.

Another common area of recurrent infections is the upper respiratory tract, especially the middle ears and sinus passages. In children, the openings are shorter and more vulnerable to the invasion of infectious organisms, which then may be hard to eradicate. It is extremely important to limit mucus-forming foods in these cases because the thick mucus greatly supports the environment necessary for pathogenic germs to proliferate. Another issue commonly missed is the ability of parasitic infections to prevent the clearance of the infection. Parasites are an important overlooked contributor to disease. Because this is a difficult subject to expose, the problems continue to escalate. It is foolish to think with all of our bare feet, all of our food bars, all of our day cares, and hospitals, nursing homes, and mass transportation, rare meats, with our poorly washed hands and toxic bodies that we do not have parasites. It is just as foolish to think that all these parasites do not cause us any harm, that it just innocently sits by and watch us thrive. We have much too much disease to assume this. We have too much resistant infections and bowel complaints to assume this. A helpful natural supplement for infections though that works very well is just to blend some honey with some garlic. You can either use fresh crushed garlic or a quality brand of powdered garlic. Place a capsule or two in a teaspoon of honey. This may be an effective anti-infective.

Another helpful treatment is to flush the nasal passages with herbal tea or even saltwater. Before using an herbal as a sinus rinse, it is good to check for allergy. Taste and smell the herb. Does it bother you? Herbal rinses can assist in sinus care. Gentle teas to use may include marshmallow root or red raspberry leaf tea. The more potent goldenseal works very well as an antibiotic wash for the nasal passages, but you can get an immediate short-lived headache after the gentle flush. Goldenseal is an extremely effective antiseptic antibacterial and may be used as a wash on all sorts of wounds. This only needs to be done once a day at most and usually only requires two or three treatments. Try to eliminate other aggravating factors. To do this, make a nice warm tea, just slightly warmer than room temperature. Place a tablespoon or so of the tea in either a bulb syringe or a special nasal irrigator, which looks like a small teapot. To understand this, do this to yourself first. Place your head sideways over the sink, hold your breath, and gently and slowly flush the tea into the upper nostril. The tea should come out the lower nostril. Some will get to the back of the throat, this you can swallow. Repeat the procedure to the other side, place head sideways, hold breath, flush another tablespoon or so of tea down the other nostril. You can repeat this a few times if there is much mucus, but with goldenseal, it only takes one treatment a day. The goldenseal will stay on the irritated lining to help limit infection. If you have a severe infection, it is best to use more benign red raspberry leaf or marshmallow root tea first, so you can tolerate the treatment better. After a treatment or two of this tea, then place the goldenseal. Again, look at the other factors contributing to the infection. Grape seed extract helps sinus passages as well and can be used topically in the nose.

Rubbing essential oil of eucalyptus on the neck and chest can also help promote expectoration as well as using a humidifier with a clean filter and water. You may also place a few drops of eucalyptus oil in the humidifier. In a few children, they may be extra sensitive to eucalyptus oil, so it might be wise to dilute the essential oil with a carrier oil such as olive or sesame or apply a small amount first to determine tolerance. I have not experienced this problem, but essential oils can be very strong, and it is always wise to dilute them first with fresh carrier oils. Don't use rancid oils here either; they do get absorbed. Smell your carrier oils; rancid oils smell bad, not fresh. It is especially important for ill children to have plenty of fresh pure air, use windows, purifiers, ionizers, and ozonators as necessary to keep your indoor air quality at its best.

Chapter 10

Digestive Complaints

Inflammatory Bowel Disease and Irritable Bowel Syndrome Identified

Inflammatory Bowel Disease (IBD) causes damage and irritation along the bowel wall. There are two primary types if inflammatory bowel disease, ulcerative colitis, and Crohn's disease. These illnesses respond to similar therapy. Many of the symptoms overlap. Ulcerative colitis causes more dilatation and thinning than Crohn's. Crohn's penetrates deeper into the tissues with inflammatory reactions. Both involve malfunctioning or autoimmune reactions with the immune system.

Crohn's	Ulcerative Colitis
1) Less obvious bleeding	1) Obvious bleeding, depending on amount and the speed at which the blood was lost red to black color (how digested darker more digested), can be very serious.
2) More deep tissue involvement, thickening of tissues	
3) Patchy involvement (cobblestone appearance)	
4) Possible fistula formation	
5) Granulomas diagnostic	2) More superficial involvement, ulcerations and erosions shallow
6) Bowel wall thickens	
7) From top to bottom possible involvement	3) Continuous involvement
8) May lead to other organ involvement with scarring and fistulas	4) No fistulas
	5) No granulomas
	6) Thinning of bowel wall
9) High risk of infection with fistulas especially	7) Involves the colon and rectum primarily
10) Pain tends to be worse and more chronic	8) Dilatation often occurs as thinning weakens wall
	9) Higher risk of free perforation due to bowel thinning
	10) UC can usually be put into remission, surgery is more helpful and permanent

In many instances you cannot distinguish one from the other completely, but in just as many you have a clear direction of the form the inflammation is going to take. Both have spasticity and griping pains, both have frustrated sufferers, and both cause chronic pain in the abdomen.

Parasites?

Think of the parasite plant mistletoe, this plant does absolutely nothing for the tree, and in fact will destroy the tree if the burden is high enough. Interestingly, certain trees such as elm are at more risk for this potentially devastating innocent looking plant. Obviously, worms and such do not look quite so innocent, but the concept is the same. Some individuals will not have the susceptibility to these invaders, or will at least not be so adversely affected, others will become quite ill, even to the point of death. Unfortunately, even though the medical texts abound on information regarding the hazards of parasites physicians do little to recognize this terrible problem do nothing to prevent it or educate patients, and do not even consider this to be a possible cause to immune problems. Parasites are devastating to the immune system. It is interesting to note cells in the blood called eosinophils marks allergy; the very same cell also marks parasites. High eosinophil counts are considered to be from "allergies", although parasites elicit the very same cellular response, in addition to other immune reactions.

Different sources of parasites include contaminated foods, bare feet on contaminated surfaces, insects, contaminated pets, and contaminated hands and other items placed in the mouth. Some parasites such as hookworms penetrate the skin. Some must enter via the mouth. Others can enter from transmission from an insect such as a flea or mosquito.

For example, there is a parasite called strongyloides that causes visceral larval migrans. The tiny worms burrow through the bowel wall and migrate. Other parasites could induce inflammatory reactions, but especially watch for strongyloides. Horses are a passion of mine, unfortunately also of strongyloides as are many domestic pets. You must treat and watch for strongyloides. In the least, a Crohn's condition would impair resistance to parasitic burdens. Strongyloides resides in the small intestine and are to a centimeter long.

—

In order to have my horses, I must diligently protect them and regularly use anti-parasitics. I recommend all pets be on an effective anti-parasite program. Also, it is important to rotate pastures on a regular basis. Herbs with antiparasitic properties include black walnut, wormwood, and turmeric, all would be useful to maintain pets as well as ourselves. The herbs must be of quality though, fresh as possible and properly prepared. Get your herbal products from reputable sources or grow them yourself. Plants produce their own natural substances that protect them from insects. These are usually considered antihelminthics (anti-worm). Adequate treatment is important. Minimize crowding and rotate the pastures. It is wise to keep the pets to an appropriate number, so the possibility of infection is lower.

Food choices and digestion

Increased mucus condition from a devitalized diet may contribute significantly to parasite burdens, as well as toxic conditions. Parasites certainly were not meant to harm us, they are a response to ignorance, crowding and ineffective immunity. Immunity is weakened from the toxicity of the contaminants in our environment and food supply. Blocking acid (from medications) is questionable because acid is our barrier to infections, and it would be much wiser to select proper foods and mind the food combining principles, chewing well. Of course acutely you must stay on the medication, but as the demand goes down, lower the frequency or dosage of medication. In time and with proper nutrition, you may need no acid-blockers at all, and have effective digestion as a result.

Any parasites could certainly make a person more vulnerable to inflammatory conditions. The immune dysfunction in genetically predisposed individuals also may make them more vulnerable to parasites as well, thus really think it out about pets with your children. Unfortunately, with the population moves, parasites will continue to become a more menacing problem that is escaping detection. Denial will only compound the issue, so be aware. Care for what your family eats. Parasites are becoming a real threat because they are dirty and unacceptable, worse than viruses. We do not like to consider them.

Other possible parasites in the activity of inflammatory bowel disease and other dysfunctional immune system reactions include tapeworms, roundworms, and hookworms. All are effectively managed by adequate treatment, diligent hand washing, keeping pets to a minimum and treated appropriately, as well as maintenance programs to prevent re-infection. Parasites can get anywhere in the body, not just the bowels. Adequate treatment requires the use of multiple herbs to minimize resistance. Using multiple herbs at the same time for 2-3 months helps manage these burdens. Maintaining good hygiene and nutrition also greatly assist. Laxatives in mild dosages may help remove the worm burden in the bowels as well, even after they have been killed. When the worms die off there can be quite an intense "die off" reaction to the debris left in your body, therefore, drinking plenty of pure water and keeping the bowels moving, eating many cleansing fruits can all help your body eliminate this burden sooner and more thoroughly.

Wash your hands frequently. Wash your children's hands frequently.

Not only care for your pets, but consider exposures from birds, rodents, and other wildlife. Under inappropriate conditions these can be sources of infection. Crowding aggravates the situation further. Birds have certain parasites of their own as well. There is a specific tuberculosis type from birds well recognized as causing lung disease, there are other fungi and parasites as well. Therefore it is very important to treat your pets effectively and regularly. Keep them hydrated and nourished. An animal with a large parasite burden may become quite ill from the die off reaction. Treatment takes more time for these animals and you must start at lower doses and go slowly to allow for recovery. Like us, animals must deal with their own "die off" reaction. In general though, your delicate little child does not need a rodent. Keep your pets cared for as children. Just be aware.

Yeasts

Yeast overgrowth with the irritation and bowel damage that occurs certainly may play a role in IBD and should be addressed. Yeasts are increasingly recognized in alternative medicine circles for their role in disease, especially inflammatory disease.

Other issues to address

Other possible causes or aggravating factors include heavy metal poisoning (such as amalgam fillings, mercury), food intolerances, and inherited predispositions. Although inheritance cannot be changed, we can make the most of what we have. Minimizing or eliminating toxins such as food contaminants and heavy metals can be of great service in restoring gastrointestinal health.

For example, the small but very significant and chronic amount of mercury released from amalgam fillings is constantly draining down the digestive tract. Mercury is a known enzyme inhibitor, and damages all tissues exposed to it. Do not allow new cavities to be filled with this toxic substance. If you can, get these out by a qualified dentist. Do only a quarter of the mouth at a time, and give plenty of time for cleansing and healing before the next set of amalgams is to be removed. Limit any swallowing of debris in the dentist chair while the amalgams are being removed. This is a costly enterprise, but well worth it for the health improvement to follow. You may experience an exacerbation of your bowel disease while your body is unloading the toxins, kelp may help as well as symptom management and cleansing activities.

Adhesions and Fistulas

Adhesions can cause partial and even complete obstruction with swelling. They can tether loops of bowel together, or attach to structures. Adhesions may be the source of female pelvic pain. Males likely get adhesions as well, but they are not as commonly detected. It is increasingly common to find adhesions during abdominal surgery even with no known risk factors such as prior surgeries or female complaints. Adhesions can be a major source of abdominal pain. Both Crohn's and ulcerative colitis sufferers get scar tissue in the form of adhesions.

Crohn's patients are more at risk for developing fistulas. Fistula involvement starts in the mucous lining or just under with ulceration. This inflammatory reaction migrates downward into the bowel wall or undermines along the intestinal lining. Penetration can occur into the muscle layers and external bowel wall. These lesions can become quite deep and penetrating. Fistulas from Crohn's sufferers can be quite long, forming canals several centimeters long. Fistulas have a significant risk of penetrating outside of the bowel wall and into other tissues, out the skin, or into organs such as the kidneys. They also can end blindly. Fistulas and adhesions are a source of much abdominal pain in Crohn's sufferers.

Both fistulas and adhesions can tether bowel loops together or to neighboring structures as well. They also can wrap around bowel loops causing narrowing of the inside of the loop. This can lead to partial or complete obstruction, depending on severity. Blind fistulas and narrowed bowel loops are especially prone to fermentation problems. These areas can become infected, a serious problem.

Yeast overgrowth with the irritation and bowel damage that occurs certainly may play a role in IBD and should be addressed. Other possible causes or aggravating factors include heavy metal poisoning (such as amalgam fillings, mercury), food intolerances, and inherited predispositions.

Bowel health can be greatly improved with natural approaches. In sufferers with any regions in the bowel that do not empty their contents regularly, either from being a blind canal or from narrowed or blocked outlets keeping the bowels loose and moving is important. Carrot juice blends can greatly help. Enemas should also be considered. As modest as we are, we should not underestimate the benefits colonic and simple enemas can have in managing these serious illnesses.

Ulcerative colitis patients do not develop the fistula canals, but certainly are at risk for developing adhesions from scar tissue.

The picture is very mixed in each individual sufferer. Bowel x-rays, barium tests, and cat scans are very limited in their ability to determine bowel problems; everything is so jumbled together. In addition, if you are self-treating, colonoscopy will be confusing to a western trained physician because of the stain from the teas, herbs, and juices. My colonoscopy exam the entire length of colon was solid black or dark brown. This confused even the most caring gastroenterologist. But I do not believe in stopping treatment to do a test to prove something, I believe in seeking health every day, especially when I am very ill. I cannot stop therapy to satisfy a test. To get an adequate diagnosis, if your symptoms are mild, you must have a high index of suspicion, you must look at the family history, and you must objectively look at the symptoms and signs.

If you are experiencing:

1) Abdominal pain that may be mild to severe depending on cause and region of involvement. The pain generally is above the organs and tissues of involvement in late disease, but in early disease the pain is usually located more in the middle of the abdomen, the "peri-umbilical" region. Abdominal pain may be the result of adhesions in the abdomen, not necessarily of bowel disease origin. For example, adhesions can cause pain in many women who have especially had children and/or any history of female problems. Adhesions are a result of scarring from any cause, so certainly surgeries to the abdomen are a source of many people's adhesions.

2) Blood in the stool, tissue in the stool (less obvious unless large amounts, looks folded and can be somewhat thin.) Mucous is different, with no real observable cellular quality and thickness. Mucous is whitish or clear. Mucous can be a symptom of colitis, whatever the cause or progression. But mucous may also be normal to some extent as well. The intestinal lining certainly does put out mucous. But for normal individuals this should be of small amount and infrequently encountered.

3) Cuts and ulcerations around the tongue, the inside of the mouth, the rectum

4) Arthralgias and other symptoms of "leaky bowel"

5) Symptoms of inflammation as in abdominal swelling and pain wherever the inflammation has set up house

6) Symptoms of fistulas that may be very subtle, with confusing discomfort at the area from affected tissues; to obvious when the fistula opens to the skin, these can become infected causing high fevers, sweats, chills, and increased pain

7) Diarrhea and bowel irritability

8) Poor appetite and intolerance to certain food and beverage substances

—

9) Granolomas—these are unusual appearing masses of various sizes that occur in the bowel wall as well as other tissues. Biopsy is necessary to confirm granuloma tissue, but many Crohn's sufferers do not get granuloma formation. They generally they resolve before the doctor appointment date is reached. Especially with self help.

10) Vitamin deficiencies from poor absorption. The terminal ileum is often involved in IBD; this is the site for Vitamin B12 for example. Other deficiencies may occur, low minerals with diarrhea, low protein with poor absorption of amino acids, and the protein building blocks.

11) Fatigue

12) Mood instability, depression and anxiety from the frustration and pain that is so commonly misunderstood, as well as possible toxins released into the blood from fermentation products within the bowel and hormonal release into the blood from bowel irritation, such as serotonin.

Think IBD.

Irritable Bowel Syndrome (IBS)

IBS involves a milder reaction with similar diverse causes, and similar symptoms including diarrhea, spasm, pain, arthralgias, and poor appetite. Irritable bowel syndrome does not have obvious physical changes such as weight loss, bleeding, and tissue alterations.

The pain in IBS can be quite debilitating though and should not be underestimated. This disease affects over 20% of the population and can cause quite debilitating symptoms that can greatly damage lifestyle quality. Although not considered deadly or as damaging, in some ways IBS is more harmful because the poor patient must be treated as a psychiatric patient

—

in the eyes of most doctors and healthcare personnel, this is unfortunate and unfair. The discouragement sufferers feel causes them to ultimately avoid getting any medical care at all, as only a few percent actually see a physician although there are literally millions of sufferers.

Fortunately there is hope. IBS responds to managing healthy bowel as in IBD. IBS in fact may be a mild IBD without the tissue damage and ulcerations, erosions, granuloma formations, and fistulas. The same causes may apply, thus the same approaches will help. Parasites and yeast overgrowth for example certainly should be addressed.

IBS is a diagnosis after you exclude the more "serious" IBD. Unfortunately, IBS being more common, it is easier to assume the problem is IBS unless you are obviously ill. Laboratory testing and imaging is very limited. There are times abnormalities are missed altogether, or are attributed to a faulty image or test. This could happen when you are treating the disease alternatively and do not look as sick as you should.

Nutritional and herbal healing can obscure the diagnosis. Realize if physicians cannot find IBD you may be doing something right. The hard thing is handling the disapproval and lack of respect for what you are doing. We just need more awareness. Stay away physicians that do not work with you, they can cause you emotional harm. We need to work together on this.

Emotional Issues

Because of the confusion about the pain and problems with eating, often those who suffer are accused of having emotional issues. I can agree, this has been an emotional issue. But we are conquerors. We are Kings and Queens. We have purpose and cause. We love and are loved. Life IS a gift, no matter how hard it may seem. So we don't understand it all now, but we are learning everyday and growing from our experiences. It is how we handle the challenges that will determine where we end up and our ultimate attitude.

The emotional issues are a reaction to the health problems as well as the fatigue, frustration, and hormonal substances released from a toxic bowel.

The liver removes toxins. If the liver is overwhelmed with clearing inflammatory debris it will not effectively clear hormones known to affect emotions. Serotonin is largely involved in bowel receptor activity, and most serotonin produced comes from the bowel. The serotonin may be released from the bowel and require this same liver deactivation or modification, as the body requires. Serotonin imbalance is implicated in many mood disorders such as anxiety and depression. Other hormones and chemicals are involved, some may not necessarily yet be recognized.

Theoretically, elevated serotonin release in the blood from the bowel may cause increased breakdown (up-regulation of breakdown function) of serotonin leading to a brain neurotransmitter deficiency. Serotonin cannot cross into the brain, there is a protective barrier preventing this. So serotonin levels in the brain may be different than the levels in the blood. The up-regulation may influence enzyme systems within the brain, causing the deficiency symptoms of depression and anxiety. Up-regulating the enzymes that break down serotonin could explain the rapid increase in depression. Many depressed patients respond well to serotonin reuptake inhibitors, which increase the available serotonin. The brain levels get too rapidly broken down while the blood levels may still be high.

The other possible role of serotonin is the bowel is using it up. In any event, IBD sufferers can respond well to therapy with mild low dose serotonin antidepressants when the disease is moderate to severe and causing depression and misunderstandings.

High serotonin levels also may be the source of some of the nausea symptoms often seen in Bowel sufferers. Serotonin in high levels certainly causes nausea, as seen in a common side effect of serotonin re-uptake

—

inhibitors, common anti-depressants, which increase the brain levels of serotonin.

Caution is advised with nausea symptoms when dealing with bowel disease and depression, use half the dose and slowly increase for therapeutic response. It is certainly a confusing picture, and serotonin alone is probably not the sole cause of the nausea seen in bowel disease sufferers. Many patients indeed respond very well to mild doses of anti-depressants that increase brain levels of serotonin, serotonin-reuptake inhibitors.

St. John's Wort may be a particularly effective alternate to serotonin-reuptake inhibitors. Historically this herb was used as a liver remedy, not an antidepressant. Since they have not truly come up with the reason St. John's Wort actually works, could it be the liver effect. In Chinese medicine the liver is the seat of emotions such as anger.

CHAPTER 11

Running on a Clean Vessel

For health and vitality, it benefits the patient, especially children who are actively growing, to keep the body pure and freely flowing in movement. Our blood is considered the river of life; this river brings nutrients to the cells and removes waste. In order for our blood to remain healthful and pure, not only do we need to take in adequate moisture, nutrients, and oxygen, but our skin, liver, lungs, bowels, and kidneys must be functioning adequately to eliminate waste products. When we are chronically exposed to excessive toxic substances, either internally generated or from external sources, these organ systems may become overwhelmed, requiring a method for storing the excesses. The liver and fat cells are two methods our body uses to store not only excess energy but also excess toxins. This is one reason it becomes so difficult to lose weight; we must allow for detoxification to eliminate unwanted fat. When we store excess toxins in the fat cells, it becomes increasingly difficult to mobilize these substances unless we improve the function of the different organs of elimination. Metabolism and energy improve as toxins get eliminated from our body; we think more clearly, and it becomes increasingly easy to incorporate further healthy practices.

It can thus be reasoned that preventing the toxic substances from building up in the first place will allow for maximum health and vitality. Our children will learn more easily and reach their maximum genetic potential. In fact, our children can ultimately do better than either parent in many circumstances because of the earlier incorporation of this understanding into the lifestyle. Us parents must do a lot of cleaning up and restoration where our children may have the advantage of getting adequate nutrition and pure foods at an earlier age. Rather than a downward trend that is usual with generational health problems, we can improve the maximum vitality our children may obtain above our own current levels. The Bible discusses generational curses, and I believe health limitations and weaknesses are a significant source of these curses. Knowledge replaces fear, as we learn to minimize the effects of our generational weaknesses. It is my sincere goal to educate, especially as many parents as possible, in healthful living practices. In this way, I hope to improve the health of future generations as much as possible rather than let the current trend of weakening health to escalate. We have so many emotional problems, early cancers, immune deficiencies, bowel disorders, and learning handicaps that plague us. As parents, we must strive to understand our own unique weaknesses as well as limitations common to most of us and incorporate this understanding into the rearing and training of our children. I believe it is an honor as well as a duty to raise emotionally, spiritually, and physically healthy children as possible in respect to our own limitations. There are certainly many parents who, out of ignorance or handicap of some sort, will not be able to provide the educational and environmental opportunities as others can. This is not necessarily their fault; it may be a product of their own upbringing and biases. But in my children's lives and in as many others as possible, my goal is to educate and enlighten. Some things may change as more truths are revealed, but the basic premise of healthful lifestyle practices cannot be underestimated.

—

Remember how the Bible discusses our body as a temple of the Holy Spirit and that we are not to defile the temple. We should not only clean the external portion of our body but also the inner portion. Regular cleansing can be easily incorporated into the lifestyles if desired. It also does not have to cost a large amount of money. In fact, although healthful foods often cost more, you will reap the rewards of less medical expenses both in the current timeframe as well as in the future. My children require very minimal antibiotics, for example. They rarely have a cold that escalates into a bacterial infection although they used to have this problem, often prior to my incorporation of active healthful practices. In addition, for example, the youngest still may get a rare ear infection: this will clear within three, at most four, days of antibiotic therapy, as opposed to the usual ten to fourteen days required. Antibiotic resistance is thwarted as immunity handles the infection better. Natural healing approaches augment medical management. Although my children have inherited a strong tendency toward allergy and asthma and have manifested these problems in the past, asthma has been eliminated and allergy is at a minimum if not completely eliminated. As my own liver has been running more purely, allergies have become much less of a problem for me when they were significantly limiting to me years ago, even with frequent exposure. Children benefit from active preventive health strategies, especially when started prenatally. They develop more fully in speech, learning, agility and growth for their potential. They may inherit constitutional weaknesses but have more building blocks to compensate with. Be aware of your child's constitution, how vital they are, and adjust for it. Find ways to maximize health. You may not have much room for error. Parents of delicate children may need ways to share their experiences. Remember not to judge others, especially when we have not had the same experiences. Realize it is our responsibility as parents to nurture our children to the best of our ability, recognizing each child has unique needs.

—

Start With the Bowel

In regard to children, be sure they are eliminating daily. Encourage them to drink plenty of healthy fluids while also encouraging intake of plenty of fresh fruits and vegetables. If necessary, use mild laxative tinctures prepared especially for children, these may include flaxseed, cascara sagrada, or turkey rhubarb. Do not use large doses, just regular small doses to prevent constipation. Apple juice also has a laxative effect, and this can help keep bowels moving freely. Fruit juices tend to be too sweet though, so it is always best to dilute the juices to 50 percent with pure water. The bowels should be moving regularly for the liver to function effectively. The liver needs a place to dump its load or it will get backed up if there is constipation. Actually, it is considered optimum to have a bowel movement after each meal. So what we as a culture consider to be "normal" for bowel movement frequency actually may not be the healthiest frequency of bowel movements. Regular daily exercise and fresh air also are helpful in relieving constipation.

On the other side of the spectrum, is when loose stools become a problem. It is still vital to get adequate fluid intake and herbal teas, especially red raspberry leaf and nettle which can go a long way, to alleviating nausea and diarrhea, especially when sweetened adequately with nutritious honey. Slippery elm gruel can help in the most stubborn and irritated cases. Not only soothing and calming, slippery elm is quite nourishing and healing to any inflamed tissues. This inner bark should be in every household for any open wounds or digestive disturbances. Keep in an airtight cool container as fresh as possible. I have applied slippery elm in one form or another hundreds of times with very reliable and well-tolerated benefits. But as a food sweetened with honey in small spoonful doses, it can be very helpful in any digestive disturbances. In cases of diarrhea in general, there is membrane barrier disturbances with potentially severe fluid shifts. Infectious, viral, bacterial, or parasitic organisms, irritant chemicals and poisons, and other various factors all may contribute to symptoms of diarrhea. It is important to get as much bowel rest as possible, getting foods that are more simple and digestible in favor of more complex foods. Here rice water and rice itself can be very helpful in restoring health. Rich cooked vegetables and vegetable broths also can be quite nourishing, supplying valuable sources of vitamins and minerals. Chicken soup certainly plays a role in many nutritious dietary approaches to diarrhea.

When the bowels are moving regularly and adequately, consider the kidneys

The kidneys, paired organs in your back, are responsible for filtering much of the blood leaving the bowel and circulating prior to its return to the liver and elsewhere. Therefore, it is important to remember to maintain kidney health at its optimum before you start with liver cleansing. Simply drinking adequate nutritive fluids and just pure water can be of tremendous aid in protecting the kidneys.

The kidneys, over time, can develop stones and other calcifications and deposits that may limit their efficiency. Drinking pure and also distilled water can not only help remove these deposits but prevent further deposition and also work to allow the deposits to be effectively eliminated. Certain herbs can help or support kidney function, think of parsley, marshmallow, oat straw, dandelion, nettle, and red raspberry leaf. By now you have learned to like red raspberry leaf tea, I hope. Small amounts of parsley can daily help to support kidney activity. Celery also would be beneficial.

When you begin the liver cleanse, waste products will be increasingly released into the bowels, possibly allowing for increased demands on the kidneys from any reabsorption that takes place. It is especially for this

—

reason it is necessary to protect your kidneys; realize everything works together.

Especially over a long period of time and without the necessary sustenance, kidneys are at risk for not only by being depleted but damaged. Kidney failure is an increasing health concern with dialysis the only option other than transplant. Please remember to support the kidneys in any healing regimen, especially for high-risk individuals such as diabetics.

To aid the kidneys in eliminating deposits, along with plenty of pure water, consider the herbs gravel root and hydrangea. These herbs promote dissolution of calcifications. Also, consider keeping a more alkaline diet, avoiding white bread and white sugar as much as possible. Red meat is also very acidifying. Parsley is also of special use in kidney disease or in preventing kidney disease. Dandelion not only aids kidney function but liver function as well. So add organic dandelions to your salads. Marshmallow root historically is a specific cure for soothing kidney structures.

Keep well hydrated. Avoid carbonated beverages. Drink nutritious herbal teas, especially red raspberry leaf and nettle. Hibiscus flowers could be quite soothing to the kidneys. More medicinal herbs for kidney health include juniper berries to promote kidney function. If you have kidney inflammation, you may want to hold or use less juniper berries in favor of more soothing herbs with anti-inflammatory properties in the kidneys. This might include hydrangea, gravel root, marshmallow, and licorice root. Use them all if you have kidney concerns while being more conservative in your use of juniper to promote detoxification. Cranberry juice has a well-known affinity for the urinary tract and can be used on a regular basis to promote kidney health. Corn silk from organic corn can also be quite nourishing to the kidneys and bladder.

When Bowels and Kidneys Have Been Addressed, Turn Attention to the Liver

After a couple of weeks of healthy bowel and kidney function, start herbs to promote liver detoxification, function, and health. Herbs in this category appropriate for child use include dandelion herb, milk thistle seed, St. John's wort, yarrow flower and herb, and barberry. Taken in regular small doses, these herbs stimulate liver cell function, bile flow, and resulting detoxification. In fact, St. John's wort historically was used as a liver alterative not an antidepressant. Many consider St. John's wort an herbal antidepressant that works for some but not others. Perhaps by clearing liver toxins, our moods improve. In Chinese medicine, the liver is highly associated with problems of anger and labile emotions. Milk thistle seed is another wonderfully useful herb; it promotes liver function as well as protects liver cells from toxic damage. Barberry root promotes liver function by stimulating bile; this not only detoxifies but promotes digestive processes. In fact, barberry is a valuable ally in managing anorexia. Anorexia relates to loss of appetite either from from digestive disturbances and toxic exposures, or from anorexia nervosa, a psychiatric disturbance. I would use barberry in anorexia nervosa as well; perhaps those affected have poor self-images because of imbalances that are poorly understood. This would not be the first "psychiatric disorder" explainable from organ imbalances. Although powerful, the mind is affected by the function or lack of function of different organs, especially the bowel, the liver, the lungs, the kidneys, the spleen, and the heart.

Most children do not have severely toxic livers, at least when they are young. If you took medications while pregnant, were in unhealthy environments while pregnant, live in a congested area, or are around chemicals such as paint and new furniture or other chemicals then liver health should be especially stressed. A manifestation of liver toxicity may be skin disorders such as psoriasis and eczema. Acne also benefits with

—

a healthy liver because the liver can efficiently process various hormones as well as other waste products in the blood for clearance. When the bloodstream is pure, which vitally requires a healthy liver, the skin will manifest this.

Kelp is also detoxifying and beneficial to the liver. Kelp is prime source of minerals as well as a scavenger of poisonous toxin from its content of alginate, an absorbent mucilage. In liver disorders with skin manifestations, include small daily doses of kelp from a reputable source.

Skin

Also, don't forget your skin as an avenue for toxin release. Promote hydration and sweating, especially with an herb such as yarrow or blessed thistle. Drink plenty of teas, even red raspberry leaf while having a hot bath to promote sweating. Also consider brushing your skin to promote this circulation. Remember it is important that we use moist heat to induce perspiration not dry. Drink as much herbal tea as possible while stimulating sweating to allow free perspiration. If severely weakened or the heart is affected, it is wise to keep a cold wet cloth over the heart region as well as address heart health. Get out of the bath slowly and wrap quickly in a dry towel. This pertains to elderly people more than children, but if you have a weakened and deficient child for whatever reason, this remedy would be easy on the heart whenever possible. Especially as the heart will work harder and be more exposed to whatever is in the blood, causing some stress response necessary for the heart. Rest after a warm bath whenever ill.

Bloodstream Cleansing

When the kidneys and liver are functioning adequately, it is good to address the bloodstream directly for cleansing purposes. As earlier stated, the blood is the river of life, and healthy blood relates to health. Supporting the blood nutritionally is important for function. Anemia can be addressed with organic sources of iron such as blackstrap molasses, alfalfa, nettle, and even red raspberry leaf herbs. Anemic children love herbal teas, sweeten to taste with honey. I do not endorse pharmaceutical iron supplements in the form of iron sulfate. I question the assimilability. Many pharmaceutical iron supplements are derived from petroleum sources, as are many less desirable vitamins. Synthetic iron supplements cause constipation in most individuals. Iron from natural sources does not cause this. Watch your sources and read your labels.

Mucus conditions affect the blood as well. As the blood gets impure plaques develop on the walls of the vessels. The heart can get quite damaged from impure blood. The degree of injury related to the specific components in the blood. Rancid and saturated and trans saturated oils all are harmful to the blood as well. Hormones and breakdown products are transported by the blood; these must be effectively cleared.

Bioflavonoids such as the soft inner peel of oranges and from various berries are especially beneficial to the bloodstream. They help to protect the vessels from toxins. Hawthorn berry is a classic example, and blueberries fall into this category. Red clover is particularly useful for blood cleansing, but when used as a tea should be combined with red raspberry and another tea for taste purposes. Red clover is a legume and has a somewhat undesirable flavor on its own. I usually combine one-two tea bags red clover with three-four red raspberry and two either hawthorn or nettle tea bags. One tea bag is approximately a teaspoon of dried herb, so if using loose herb, substitute teaspoons for bags. Children will more readily drink the tea, especially when sweetened to taste, honey ideally. Herbal

—

teas are especially effective for children. Elderberry is another tea that is strong on its own but combines well in the base tea above. This herb is rich in bioflavonoids as well.

Juices, especially carrot and beet juice, are particularly cleansing. Grape juice is a very well tolerated blood cleanser that may or may not need to be diluted depending on your situation. Fresh carrot juice combined with either celery or beets does a wonderful job in supporting the blood. In severe cases, you may want to let the juice warm up a little to room temperature. This places less work on the digestive system. Let the juice warm in the mouth before swallowing. An old saying is to "fletcherize," meaning to chew thoroughly even your juice. Drink more slowly though when ill and deficient.

Garlic can help the blood by providing beneficial sulfur moieties that are effective reducing agents, important for detoxification functions. Garlic also is especially anti-infection. Use some caution because garlic may be too hot in large doses for delicate or weakened individuals. So determine tolerance before jumping to large doses.

In dosing children with herbs consider this approach. A child two-six would require approximately one-fourth the dose of an adult. The six-twelve age group would get half the dose. Twelve and up can generally get a full herbal dose, depending on the size of the child to some extent. Give them a "small" adult dose. Usually labels on reputable herbs give very conservative and safe doses although they may not be absolutely complete. The mild acting more nutritive herbs such as nettle, red raspberry, catnip, and hawthorn teas are very safe. There are only rare allergic reactions and intolerances to any herbs. A young child usually can tolerate well one crushed clove of garlic in honey or one capsule of powdered garlic. To use garlic as a supplement take once a day for anti-infection purposes increase the garlic dose to at least three times a day.

—

A review of febrile infections

Fever can help the body clear itself from infections and other damaging exposures when in a controlled fashion; with moist heat, the body gets a chance to flush toxins and wastes and destroy organisms. When you have fever, you may want to cover both the head and the heart of the child with moist cool towels, depending on the degree of physical response and constitution of the child. When your child is ill, it is better to take the child off foods and encourage herbal teas adequately sweetened, best with honey. When the child does eat, make the foods simple and easily digestible. Of course, keep sugars and white flour though to a minimum. White sugar and white flour impair the immune system. An acute viral infection often elicits an acute fever that requires competent care. It is especially important to maintain hydration in high fevers. Sometimes in these cases, I would use a pharmaceutical medication such as Tylenol or Advil. This is especially necessary when the child is very uncomfortable. Fevers should not be allowed to be dry. Hydration helps patients tolerate any fever. A few sips at a time, soothing teas and medicines often are sufficient to control a fever. Get control of the fever even if it takes pharmaceuticals as keeping hydration is cornerstone to healing. Gently encourage herbal teas at room temperature or slightly warmer. Cool herbal teas requires energy to bring the tea to body temperature but if they are tolerated they can be used. They may be unnecessary stress and work to the ill body. You can wash the child down though with moist cool washcloths. But do not chill the child.

CHAPTER 12

Detoxification

The purpose of detoxification is to allow your body to flush out impurities and waste matter that has gotten lodged in tissues. Heavy metals, chemicals, and devitalized food all lead to conditions of toxic buildup. The buildup occurs throughout the body, some toxins have specific predilections sometimes determined by old injuries, genetic risks, and vulnerable sites. For example, mercury tends to accumulate in the pituitary. Mercury also accumulates in the kidneys. This heavy metal is monitored by the ADA and the FDA but should not be considered safe in any amount. Amalgam fillings, composed of up to half mercury, slowly release mercury into the blood and gastrointestinal tract; the mercury here blocks multiple normal enzymatic functions for cell life.

How rapid we detoxify varies to the individual. If you are strong and healthier you can handle a faster detoxification treatment. If you are weak and deficient you must go slower in your detoxification.

Detoxification uses fasts, herbs, pure water, steam baths, towel rubs, sweat lodges, meditation, and exercise to help the body clear itself of accumulated toxic debris.

Juicing is particularly useful and detoxifies even when you are not using the juice for the purpose. Juicing is one of the best-known detoxification treatments. Get a quality juicer. In some health food stores, you can purchase carrot juice bottled; but because it is not as fresh, it is lacking much of the active enzymes fresh carrot juice has. These enzymes are helpful in digestion. You can mix carrot juice with celery juice, beet juice, parsley juice, or even apple juice for a great fasting juice. Another easy fasting juice is grape juice, Welch's is likely the safest brand if you do not juice the grapes fresh.

A blood transfusion could be made out of carrot juice five pounds with beet juice, three large roots, and parsley or dandelion for mineral and chlorophyll value (or chlorophyll itself) and half the amount of beets. In deficient individuals, drink juice rather slowly to allow full salivation and chew until very watery, "Chew your juice." Celery is also excellent in juice preparations due to the calcium and especially silica content necessary for proper calcium utilization.

There also herbs important to most detoxification regiments to help the process along and also help protect the body from reacting to toxins released from stored places back into the blood. These stored toxins may be saccharin, cadmium, mercury, waste matter from putrefactive bacteria, food additives and preservatives such as benzoic acid, and others from artificial vitamins. Poor vitamins are worse for you than good for you because of the toxins they may harbor.

Eating wholesome foods goes a long way in keeping toxins at bay, also exercise and plenty of fresh water.

If you happen to need to lose weight, detoxification is a must if you want permanence. Toxins are often stored in fat to keep them from causing harm. Rapid weight loss causes much muscle breakdown but also causes much toxin release from fat cells. This can be very uncomfortable. People will believe that the herbs have caused the problem or the symptoms are just coincidental. These toxins, especially for weight problems, need gentle regular release. You will get to a healthier weight simply by detoxifying.

Simple Methods for Detoxification

1. Juicing
2. Drinking plenty of pure water to avoid dehydration and encourage elimination
3. Grapefruit before breakfast in the morning
4. Prune juice first thing in the morning
5. Herbal supplements
6. Enema treatments
7. Exercise
8. Sweating
9. Deep Breathing
10. Good attitudes
11. Adequate rest

Organ Specifics

For more thorough detoxification, it is important to approach this orderly as previously mentioned.

1. Bowels first

Start with getting the bowels moving. The bowels must be moving adequately in order for the liver to unload toxins effectively and safely. Prune juice in the morning is a good start. Adequate pure water intake and magnesium as a supplement encourage safe bowel activity.

Herbal laxatives may be useful for any detoxification method and are usually quite effective. They stimulate as well as nourish the bowel. Detoxifying herbs that encourage bowel activity include cascara sagrada, bitternut, turkey rhubarb, senna, and aloe vera. These herbs nourish the bowel lining as they stimulate function. They should be used in dosages necessary to encourage two-three bowel movements daily. Decrease the dosage as the need for the herbal supplements goes down. This is evidenced by increased sensitivity to the herbal laxatives. Keep the diet as healthy as you can while you are doing this; do not rely on herbs to substitute for a bad diet.

Herbal enemas also may be quite helpful in allowing the bowels to be restored to their normal function. Enemas should be done every other day to once a week for detoxification purposes to six weeks duration.

As the bowel musculature heals through good nutrition and the removal of offending foods, the muscle tone improves and the need for herbal laxatives decreases naturally. Mucus forming foods such as white flour and white sugar products, as well as dairy products, can be quite detrimental in bowel cleansing and function and should be avoided. Flaxseed and other beneficial oils on the other hand can be quite nourishing and supportive to bowel health. Also, fruits and vegetables offer valuable fiber sources that encourage healthy bowel function. Figs are especially nutritive.

2. Skin (Can begin at any time)

Hot bathes with plenty of herbal teas helps o open pores allowing detoxification out the skin. The skin is quite effective in releasing toxins when allowed to with perspiration from heat and exercise. Avoiding aluminum containing antiperspirants is important in allowing these important avenues of detoxification to function at their optimum. This

—

may be why breast cancer is on the rise or at least one of the reasons being aluminum is so prevalent in our society, as is breast cancer in both men and women.

There are many alternative deodorants and antiperspirants that are effective when used regularly. Crystal salts are quite effective when used regularly and seem much less harmful. These are widely available in health food stores and lasts for several months at the least. Natural deodorants also are widely available with combinations including lavender, tea tree oil, and others being quite helpful in masking odor.

After stopping aluminum containing antiperspirants, it is necessary to take as many as two or three bathes a day for two or three weeks if possible to avoid odor. Your body is releasing toxins that have been stored for quite a while. After a couple of weeks though, you will find the need for bathing to diminish as your body, especially your liver, runs in a cleaner state.

Dry brushing and toweling after a hot bath also helps the skin to breathe. Herbs useful for diaphoretic effects drunk in tea form include yarrow, hyssop, and blessed thistle. Red raspberry tea also has mild diaphoretic properties and should be added for flavor at least. These teas are especially useful when taking hot bathes to avoid dehydration. Dry heat is dangerous, moist heat is healing as well as stimulating to the immune system.

3. Kidneys

It is important to support the kidneys as you are detoxifying; the kidneys have delicate structures that can be greatly be harmed by the rapid elimination of toxins without protection. This again stresses the need for adequate hydration by drinking pure water. Herbal teas and fruit juices are also useful for maintaining hydration, especially grape and cranberry juice.

Herbs for kidney support include dandelion, marshmallow root, hydrangea root, gravel root, juniper berries, and herbs that support circulation in general including but not limited to hawthorn berry, blueberries, ginkgo, gotu kola, cayenne, and pau d'arco.

4. Liver

A healthy and well functioning liver is paramount to maintaining a pure bloodstream. The liver is one of the most important organs for the processing and elimination of toxins as well as the production of building materials such as proteins to maintain renewal. Thus with all the toxic exposure in our environment, what we are eating, breathing, drinking, etc., the liver is increasingly in high demand.

The liver has three known methods for detoxification that involves making toxins and other wastes soluble in water and/or adequately washed out of the body.

To support all three phases of liver function, provide plenty of pure water for optimum circulation. Use herbs, supplements, and foods with high sulfur content, such as garlic and MSM, to naturally support conjugation of toxins. Many widely available herbs such as barberry, gentian, yellow dock, and dandelion encourage healthy liver activity. Also, many nutraceuticals, concentrated nutrients, are now available such as alpha-lipoic acid that may be especially useful for all phases of detoxification. In general, bitter herbs and foods support liver detoxification activity, so regularly include bitters in your diet.

It is important that the liver is functioning well and all pathways are supported before you undertake blood detoxification. Phase 2 detoxification pathways need to be supported to manage toxic byproducts of the phase one pathways. If these issues are not addressed, the liver may be hit with too much toxicity too rapidly, leading to liver irritation and possibly liver damage.

The appropriate supportive foods and herbs, along with a healthy lifestyle along with adequate pure water intake, can usually prevent this injury.

5. Blood

After you have been supporting the cleansing organs one or two weeks or more depending on your starting point—how much toxins you suspect to be harboring—work on blood cleansing. Determine your risks by how much fat you are carrying, how much junk food you eat, the air and water quality you are exposed to, and other lifestyle habits. If you have acne, blood cleansing is especially warranted as the liver is having trouble detoxifying hormones as well as toxins and is overwhelmed.

The skin is an outward manifestation of the health of the blood. Hair and nails also can suggest this, as well as the brightness of the eyes. The blood is the "river of life." When the blood is impure, all tissues are affected. When the blood is fresh and pure, the tissues manifest this as well. Saying this, the blood is paramount in kidney, heart, brain, liver and all other organ health. This is why smoking is so absolutely harmful. Not only do you get the vasoconstriction (constricted blood vessels) of the nicotine, you get all the toxins from pesticides to additives from the tobacco. It is no wonder smoking is attributed to all kinds of cancer and clotting risks.

Pure blood is more alkaline; the pH is slightly higher. When we are ingesting acidic foods such as white flour and white sugar products, we are increasing our cancer risk. It is well recognized in alternative cancer approaches to alkalinize the body with "potassium broth" and other healthful vegetables steamed lightly. Alkalinizing the blood, and therefore the body, discourages cancer. This is so very poorly understood in Western medicine but is the basis of much of the successful cancer alternative therapies around the world. Body acidity can be indirectly determined by the urinary pH in general, the lower the number the more acidic. Salivation should be encouraged with adequate healthful fluid intake as well as thorough chewing. Saliva is naturally alkaline. Drinking lemon water and eating salads including bitter greens stimulates salivation as well. Also, this could be why so many have trouble with acidic foods such as orange juice; they may already be having trouble with an acidic condition.

Anyway, after you have been off the carbonated beverages and other toxic artificial "foods" and been eating plenty of ideally organic vegetables and fruits, there are herbs you can add to encourage blood cleansing. These include red raspberry leaves, as you might expect. Red raspberry leaves are very mild and safe and should be in the home of every family. Other valuable blood cleansing herbs include blessed thistle leaves, red clover blossoms and leaves, burdock root, sarsaparilla root, and garlic. Chaparral leaves also are quite cleansing to the blood but very powerful and should be monitored by a competent physician.

Distilled water, which is "empty water," is especially useful for blood cleansing and is quite capable of removing inorganic mineral deposits from arterial walls and other deposits. The water should be followed though with adequate organic mineral intake, such as the minerals available in blackstrap molasses and alfalfa leaves. Be aware that alfalfa leaves do thin blood. Molasses and kelp do not. In this way, you substitute useless inorganic, inassimilable minerals for alkalizing organic, assimilable minerals over a period of time. Distilled water, as previously mentioned, is quite useful in preparing herbal teas as it extracts up to 30 percent more of the nutrients from the herbs than regular purified water.

Burdock root, for example, has a long history of being useful in acne management. The other blood cleansers would apply as well, as long as the diet is appropriate and the other organs have been addressed.

—

Side Effects

As you are undergoing a cleansing routine, you will experience discomfort as toxins are being released into the blood and then out of the body. If this is intolerable, you must slow down your cleansing process and increase the amount of time you spend in your cleanse. You also should be getting adequate rest, keep your agenda to a minimum, and exercise regularly as tolerated to encourage circulation. You can also take supportive herbs and foods such as hawthorn berry, berries in general, carrots and celery, leafy green vegetables, ginkgo leaves, cayenne fruit in low doses, and catnip leaf.

After the cleansing process, you will notice weight loss as the toxins no longer require places for their storage, more energy and stamina, and better sleep quality. Your hormones should be better balanced, as your liver health is improved and now able to manage the hormone load for detoxification. You should be less vulnerable to infections and illness in general, and your vitality should be improved tremendously without the need for artificial stimulants such as caffeine. Your mood should be stable and positive, as the negative emotions are released from a healthier liver. All of this though may require more than one cleansing routine; you may have much to unload and should not try to do it all in one cleansing cycle. In many references, it is suggested you cleanse twice a year, once in spring and once in fall. This to me is sound advice.

CHAPTER 13

Symptom Management

In affected adults, the spouse, loved ones, and children, all must learn to be patient, helpful, and caring. These are trying times for them as well. Because of the way this disease manifests during such a prime time in a person's life, often in the twenties and thirties, there is guilt because the sufferers no longer can do what they could before and may have children and others counting on them when the illness manifests.

When the disease affects children, mood fluctuations and poor eating habits frustrate the problem. Super nutrition in the form of supplements of fresh, wholesome foods, whole food concentrates, beneficial oils, and nourishing herbs may tremendously help your child grow and mature. Good diet greatly benefits any child, as well as incorporating in it nourishing herbs. Ample red raspberry leaf tea blends is nourishing and calms any nausea the child may be suffering from. These children may develop physical and emotional growth delays, as they are malnourished if left unchecked by ignorance, pride, or severity of disease. Nutrition is paramount in children always, and supplements can greatly aid these children in recovery and vitality.

Caution

When you have mild bowel symptoms or moderate ones that have not been clinically identified and you effectively manage your own disease, you might be accused of malingering. Malingering is a term used for those who use illness for attention. Sufferers should to be trying to get better to their abilities, not complaining and only wanting medications to control symptoms. By striving for wellness, we are not malingering. Laxatives used in therapy may be harmful to some, but we must still strive to educate ourselves and others of their safe usefulness. When you are faced with misunderstandings, don't take this personally and realize it is ignorance, culture, and possibly even arrogance that are at fault.

People who do not suffer these illnesses cannot understand the frustration, the pain, the confusion and other aspects of a disease that generally hits at the prime of a person's life, sometimes completely unexpected, sometimes with some "red flags" that had been ignored. So please do not fault these well-meaning doctors that inescapably judge. They have been trained to evaluate things, as they do this in their daily healing. With all their education and training, herbal wisdom has been lost in traditional medicine. It needs to be brought back safely.

People who go to medical school tend to have more mental and physical stamina to meet the intense demands. They may not be able to empathize with more delicate individuals until they mature in their experiences. Few people who go to medical school suffer from health handicaps. Until you understand fully, it is hard to empathize. It may become frustrating only because of lack of understandings. We all have room to grow. Fortunately there are sympathetic doctors.

Many autoimmune syndromes affect people in their prime, their 20s to 30s. Men, who get these diseases less frequently, may choose less demanding positions and may self-medicate to cover their problems. Women may also respond this way. In addition, women tend to start babies or professions in these same twenties and thirties, so their symptoms tend to be exacerbated with the demands of pregnancy or other stress.

Finding a doctor, male or female, who really understands IBD is difficult but they are out there. We are learning. So realize where they are at, and tell them what they need to know as you learn to trust their management and they learn to help you manage this illness. Don't go for the latest drugs or surgeries unless you are in an emergency. Try to keep both intestines and intestinal function as long as possible. Work together, the gastro specialist has room to learn as well. Realize colonoscopies show herbal stain as well as illness, and this can be new for the doctor performing the colonoscopy. New does not mean bad, and change can come. He was able to say things looked ok or not.

Those herbs had likely saved my life during that time and times since. Usually though, I do not get into life-threatening inflammation before I am starting therapies that have been effective specific to whatever symptoms I am experiencing. The goal is to stop symptoms and improve vitality and immunity, but this takes a step at a time. The bigger goal is to not allow this illness to rob your life of meaning and hope, to minimize permanent damage, and live fully functional vital lives. Use your own judgment with guidance from a physician who respects your attempts at wellness. Do not let yourself get caught in an ego game but find another doctor that suits you better. Also, appreciate your doctors suggestions and viewpoint.

The symptoms of bowel disorders often overlap, so they will be considered together. Because IBD tends to cause more severe symptoms, I will refer to this disease entity more exclusively, but the same remedies would apply for any bowel sufferers.

1. Anorexia (loss of appetite)

The anorexia stems from multiple causes. For instance, as a person realizes eating equals pain, even subconsciously, he or she starts to avoid

—

eating. Over time, the stomach shrinks, limiting the intake of food. Also, since the dysfunctional bowel is releasing toxins into the blood, the sufferer may feel somewhat poisoned; as the liver is unable to handle the demand. The liver is flooded with extra hormonal, putrefactive, and inflammatory byproducts, as well as the wastes it normally handles. Helping to heal the liver and support liver function with nourishing liver herbs, supplements, and gentle regular detoxification practices, is important in the effective management of IBD to improve appetite. The late Dr. Christopher recommended barberry specifically for anorexia. Barberry is a major liver remedy.

2. Motility problems

A. Constipation

Constipation is poorly tolerated, especially in those sufferers of IBD. You cannot have distension and accumulation of waste without consequences. This must be addressed in a safe and effective manner. As you restore bowel function with nutritive laxatives such as cascara sagrada that tonify and strengthen bowel musculature, you will eventually require fewer laxatives. If you use pharmaceutical type laxatives, for example, ex-lax or phenylpthalein (BAD), all you are doing is pushing the bowels without strengthening them and nourishing them. This is similar to taking stimulants, you are pushing the system without addressing the underlying issue or nourishing the affected tissues that have become so sluggish.

Natural laxatives are not addictive physically for when they are used appropriately they should tone and nourish the bowels. These herbs must be used appropriately in bowel complaints. Ultimately, you require less laxatives of herbal origin as your body gets more toned and strengthened. This is not always the case, but is usually the case.

—

Now if you have adhesions and partial obstructions, herbal laxatives may play a special role. With partial obstructions, the risk is for the bowel to completely close off. Keeping the food in a slightly loose consistency as stool is important for it to navigate the bowel through the narrowed passages. First using proper foods, occasional laxatives help stimulate bowel activity and keep the bowels moving loose. Laxatives should not be used for severe symptoms, as you do not want to use them on completely obstructed bowels. We should keep the stool somewhat loose if we are at risk for blockage. Treat preventively. Over time the herbs can restore function. With regular use of herbal tonic laxatives, you become more sensitive to laxatives. After years of feeding the bowel tissues with proper tonic laxatives and good nutrition with foods, supplements, and herbs the bowels will likely move regularly on their own.

One particular herb deserves mention as it has so effectively restored bowel function and is not a laxative. This herb is mullein or *Verbascum thapsus*. This amazing herb has healed the digestive tract to such a degree that laxatives are now only occasionally required, and absorption of nutrients has been restored as well. I also believe the herb has been restoring immune function in general, and historically the herb is known as a "glandular." Mullein also is greatly restorative to the lungs. Wild mullein has been considered nature's toilet paper with its' big soft leaves.

Total obstruction or blockage leads to surgery if not reversed in enough time. Keeping the bowels inflammation down and movements loose prevent against obstruction. You especially take care of what you eat. Avoid pizza, nuts, seeds, breads. Take juices. Teas, gentle foods and herbs all calm irritation helping it pass. Early awareness can help you prevent worsening blockage. Stay hydrated.

Minimizing surgery can go a long way in maintaining vitality; having the bowel cut out is not always a quick fix. You then have no chance of restoring the function of the bowel lost from the knife. On the other hand, if the tissue is dead, surgery may provide you with great hope and

—

improved vitality with much less pain. But if there is a chance at restoring the tissue, take it.

Herbs with laxative, tonic, alterative, and nutritive value include cascara sagrada, turkey rhubarb, senna, and butternut. Senna and turkey rhubarb are used in formulas for children, often combined with peppermint or ginger. Young children can be especially vulnerable to constipation but usually do not get obstructive symptoms until later in life. Mullein again has particularly nutritive benefit to the digestive system.

Do not use pharmaceutical laxatives with no tonic or nutritive value.

Cascara sagrada and turkey rhubarb are safe when used modestly and improve intestinal tone supporting the tissues. Magnesium is helpful for improving bowel frequency and is quite safe and healthful. Most people, especially those who have been on white flour/white sugar diets, are magnesium deficient. This mineral is necessary for many functions, including nervous actions. Flaxseed can be laxative for patients but should be used in care for those with obstructive symptoms. You do not want a lot of bulk in a narrow canal. Flaxseed oil can be used alternatively, and it not only provides some laxative properties but also provides valuable nutrition and anti-inflammatory action.

Some herbs are mildly laxative such as licorice, mullein and dandelion. Herbs that are used to stimulate bile flow, such as barberry, will also help. Bile itself has a laxative effect, and stimulating the liver has the added benefit of eliminating toxin loads.

Drinking plenty of pure water is important for bowel health habits as well as other health reasons. Purify the water though by a quality water filtering system for your home and change the filters regularly.

Do not ever use castor oil for laxative purposes; this is very toxic to delicate mucous membranes. Mineral oil is milder but still not nutritive and impairs absorption of other nutrients such as good fats. I do not recommend this either.

Feed your bowels. Glutamine and glycine and N-acetyl-glucoseamine are all bowel-lining foods. Butyrate also is nutritional for inner bowel lining and is available in butter. If your bowel is poorly functioning, in addition to gentle laxatives, encourage healing with these supplements. Slippery elm as gruel or in a shake is quite nutritive to bowel tissues and is invaluable as a source of nutrition for the bowel. Mullein and marshmallow root are similarly nutritious and healing for bowel lining. Licorice root is invaluable in inflammatory bowel as in any inflammatory condition but should be used with care.

B. Spasticity

When the bowel is irritated, over-distended, or even inflamed and ulcerating, the muscles react with spasm. This can be quite uncomfortable, even painful with "griping" cramps. This is especially painful when there is one or more partial obstructions the spasms are slamming against. Crohn's sufferers with their thickened bowel walls are less at risk for perforation than ulcerative colitis, which causes bowel wall thinning, although this does happen. Thin bowel wall increases risk of perforation, and this is deadly. So keep the distension at a minimum with a responsible diet, gentle herbal laxatives, control inflammation, and use of anti-spasmodic herbs, and other therapies below as necessary.

Herbs

Antispasmodic herbs are very safe. They also are quite effective. The best known is peppermint. The plant leaves can be made into a tea, and enteric-coated capsules of peppermint oil are available in most health food stores that allow the peppermint oil to be released into the small bowel directly. Other valuable, safe antispasmodic herbs include red raspberry leaf, ginger, and catnip.

Teas

Teas are prepared quite simply. It is important to use purified or distilled water. Distilled water has the added benefit of being empty in constituents, so distilled water pulls out the medicinal qualities more effectively than regular purified water, according to qualified sources, by up to 30 percent more efficiency at pulling out nutrients and medicinal constituents. The main thing to remember though is to only drink water that is purified adequately; we are adding too many substances and toxins into our "drinking" water supply on tap.

A tea blend can be quite calming and is easily tolerated. I use a base of red raspberry leaves (1/3), and add nettle leaves (for nutrition and anti-inflammatory action), catnip leaves (calming), peppermint leaves (antispasmodic), wood betony leaves (nervine and antispasmodic), lemon balm leaves (nervine and antispasmodic), and valerian root (antispasmodic and nervine) if you can tolerate the smell. You do not need to use all these, just two or three in addition to the red raspberry leaf. Find what works for you. The red raspberry leaf when gathered and dried appropriately is flavorful and makes the medicinal tea taste good with or without honey.

Herbal supplements are available in multiple ways. The tinctures are often in alcohol, which should be avoided unless you are using minute amounts for specific reasons. Glycerin tinctures, prepared for children primarily, can be of great use for spasm. Look at all the colic blends available. In these blends, look for the above herbs as well as skullcap, black cohosh, lobelia (in small amounts is anti-spasmodic), and fennel (for associated gas). Powders in capsules and tablets also may be of help.

—

Choose quality over quantity. Smell the powder inside the capsule except valerian.

Not only address the spasms with medicinal herbs but also look around your lifestyle. Are you being overly stressed? Do you get enough rest? Are you worrying too much? All these can add to the spastic reactions. Calm yourself; rebalance your life by facing priorities and removing drains.

Moist heat also is of tremendous benefit for spasms. Use a pack made for back pain or hot water bottle on your abdomen to increase circulation, take a hot bath while drinking plenty of fluids.

Massage, gently done, can also calm spasticity. Massage calms the mind, which can greatly help to calm to bowels. The mind is intricately connected to many organs, especially the bowels and the heart.

A gentle massage to the abdomen with castor oil has been quite helpful in relieving spasms. Castor oil stimulates immune function as well as helps to dissolve calcifications and adhesions. Olive oil and wheat germ oil also can be used and are quite nourishing.

Gentle, therapeutic high enemas help with spasticity. Use the same medicinal herbs as in the tea above. Slightly warm gentle, slow enemas can greatly alleviate the pain and griping spasms cause. You can tolerate some herbs better this way, such as valerian (you do not have to taste or smell it). Marshmallow root can be blended into the enema tea for much healing relief. Marshmallow has the added benefit of nourishing and protecting the kidneys as well as the intestinal lining. Slippery elm in small amounts can be blended into the enema tea. Blend well with an electric blender to adequately thin the fluid so it will run freely through the enema tubing.

How To Do a Safe Enema

You must make a quality tea; bitter herbs work very well in enema fluids as bitters stimulate liver function better than any other flavor. Bring pure water, either well filtered or distilled, to a boil; add approximately 6 teaspoons of tea to 1-1 1/2 quarts of water. Simmer until slightly warmer than room temperature, mild bathwater temperature may be fine. If the tea is in bag form, remove the bags; if the tea is loose, filter out the rough material. Pour the tea into a blender and add marshmallow root, slippery elm, licorice root, or any other powders you might want to include. Blend well. Add more pure water to meet temperature and dilution requirements. The fluid must flow easily through the enema tubing.

Herbs you might consider are the following:

1. Catnip
2. Hyssop, bitter, milder than yarrow, and antiseptic as well.
3. Peppermint (antispasmodic)
4. Yarrow can be sensitizing for some as it is a cousin of ragweed, is particularly bitter and useful for liver health.
5. Milk thistle for liver support
6. Red raspberry leaf is gentle, astringent, and nourishing.
7. Dandelion
8. Plantain
9. Ginger, peel off bark of fresh root, strip into slices, place in the tea and strain out matter after the tea has simmered and cooled.
10. Licorice root in tea form, the powder can be added to the blender.
11. Marshmallow root can be used in tea or powder form.
12. Slippery elm is not available as a tea, but the powder certainly should be blended in the enema fluid after the tea has simmered and cooled.
13. Garlic in small amounts can be blended in although it can be quite stimulating to the bowel. Garlic is very healing and stimulating but should be used with care in enemas for its stimulating effects to tissues.

14. Organic coffee is used alone; it does not need other herbs for the cleansing and detoxifying effect. Like attracts like, coffee in enema form effectively causes the liver to dump toxins into the bowel to be eliminated.

15. White oak bark helps strengthen bowel tissues.

*

You can purchase enema materials at any drugstore; look for a hot water bottle, an enema bag, or a vaginal douche bag, these may be the names used. Keep this equipment in a private and safe place.

First of all, it is very important your equipment be clean and the tip of the enema tube be well lubricated. The fluid should be slightly warm; if it is too hot, it could be damaging to the intestinal lining as well as very difficult to keep in for medicinal action. If it is too cold, it may cause some spasm and thus limit the flow but is generally easier to retain for medicinal action.

After the enema tea is prepared and placed in a standard hot water bottle/enema (vaginal douche) bag, place it on the bathroom counter at about the height of the doorknob. Never force the fluid into you, let it gently run in by gravity alone. Never force anything. Place one or two towels under you for comfort, use one to cover yourself. When first learning to do enemas and when very ill, always have a loved one available, not necessarily in the same room, but available to help.

*

Lie first on your left side, and gently insert the tip of the tube into your rectum. Gently massage your abdomen and let some of the tea flow in as tolerated. Stop the flow when you become uncomfortable. After a while, go to the toilet and allow this to evacuate. Then repeat the process, lying on your left side and allowing the tea to flow into your bowel. Gently massage the fluid upward toward your left shoulder in your abdomen. Let this sit a while and be patient. If necessary go to the toilet to evacuate but try to go slow enough that the medicinal tea can help.

As the enema proceeds, you may feel lightheaded or nauseous as toxins are released into the bloodstream. This is why it is so important to go slow and only do a small amount at a time. After a few treatments, you will not be releasing so many toxins and will be able to tolerate higher enema treatments.

As you progress in this therapy, you will repeat the above, introducing the tea into the left side as before. Then you can rise onto your knees with your bottom in the air. Gently massage the fluid across your abdomen from left to right and rest here a while. Slow the flow as needed to tolerance. After a short while shift over to your right side and allow the fluid to descend into the right side of your colon to your appendix and cecum. This completes a "high" enema. Gently massage as you can. Go slow. Evacuate as necessary. After you have rested in this position as long as you can tolerate, finish your evacuation. Rest as needed to recover from any toxins released.

You will feel so much better after a few adequate treatments. Nausea, allergies, and liver disease all can be greatly relieved with this technique over time. For liver function, you might add hyssop tea to your enema fluid. Yarrow is also cleansing to the liver but can be quite strong and even irritating for some.

During the enema therapy, it may be comfortable to massage some castor oil on the abdomen, as previously mentioned, for spasticity.

*

Fluids absorbed from the colon enter the liver and the kidney systems for organization and detoxification. When you use enemas with medicinal value, much of the fluids absorbed go to the liver and some to the kidneys. The circulation is such that bitter herbs can greatly improve liver function and health by enema form. The herbs have are quickly and more completely brought to the liver in this way.

*

Get adequate exercise as you can tolerate. Start low and go slow. Movement stimulates circulation that can effectively help healing. Be careful not to overdo it; you will pay the price in increased inflammation and pain. The increased inflammation inevitably wears you out. Be persistent though, but do less than you think you can rather than more. With autoimmunity, it is very important to keep moving and living actively but also very important not to overdo it. There is a fine balance.

I look at these diseases as a way to stay away from the wrong things and stay with good lifestyle choices. Diseases have a way of doing that. For example, diabetics must learn a better diet; IBD sufferers must learn an extreme level of balance in their lifestyle in addition to diet. Think of disease as keeping you out of trouble.

C. Diarrhea

Diarrhea can be quite troublesome. This generally results from the bowel irritation and inflammation and poor absorption capabilities. Using medicinal foods and herbs can greatly improve bowel function, such as with absorption. To help assuage diarrhea, use gentle foods and herbs that are extremely easy to digest. Nourish, nourish, nourish. Here again, slippery elm gruel is profoundly effective. Slippery elm also can be added to a nutritional shake. The powder is so mucilaginous, you must blend vigorously to get the herb to dissolve, as previously mentioned; using an electric blender can be helpful. You must add the powder in gradually or it will fly everywhere. Remember this for enemas, slippery elm may be added to the warm tea made for enema; use by blending a small amount in it after the tea has been prepared. Slippery elm is the inner bark of the red elm tree, an endangered plant. Marshmallow root and mullein might be an alternative or an addition to slippery elm used in capsule, tea, or enema preparations. These plants are not completely equivalent though, so grow red elm trees whenever you can. These cannot be replaced. Plantain as a powder or supplement may also help diarrhea problems by allowing for healing of the intestinal lining.

Address provoking factors: yeasts, pathogenic bacteria, viruses, and parasites, all often resulting from putrefaction

Yeasts may cause bowel irritation leading to diarrhea. Address this issue if you are at risk. There are several helpful yeast syndrome books that are available, and this is an increasing problem with all the antibiotics, birth control pills, and sugar diet. Lessen your yeast burden. This yeast I am speaking about is overgrown in the bowels and can escape into the blood to become systemic. Yeasts cause all kinds of symptoms, on top of the list though is muscle pain, sugar cravings, bowel irritation, and food sensitivities. One pill of pharmaceutical medicine though will not cure a yeast syndrome; this takes months and is a long-term follow through. If you do not keep up with the yeasts, they will become a problem again.

As traditional physicians, we may underestimate the yeast problem. Just because you do not have vaginal yeast does not mean you do not have systemic yeast. But if you do have recurrent vaginal yeast infections, you most definitely have a yeast problem. Address it. After a month of treatment, or even sooner, you will notice much improvement of your health by following an anti-yeast protocol. There is a pharmaceutical medication that is quite helpful in destroying yeasts, thus reducing the sugar cravings that allow the yeasts to be fed and multiply. Yeasts cause symptoms of hypoglycemia as they rob you of your blood sugar.

Herbs and supplements also help manage and even eliminate yeast overgrowth situations. These include mullein, black walnut, caprylic acid, and probiotics such as lactobacillus. Caprylic acid works by enzyme action against the yeast cell wall. Acidophilus and similar probiotics help by taking up space in the bowel and pushing the yeasts "out." They should be started low and gradually increased to avoid gas pain from adding too many bacteria at a time. Probiotics also help to manage parasite issues.

Avoiding sugar foods can help but may be almost impossible if the yeasts are already a problem. Use herbs or appropriate pharmaceuticals as determined by a knowledgeable physician to destroy the yeasts, and the cravings for sweets will literally go away. Yeast overgrowth certainly worsens sugar cravings. If your cravings for sugary foods go away with yeast treatments, suspect this as a component to your health situation.

Parasites may play a role in diarrhea conditions as well. They irritate and inflame the inner bowel. The acid in the stomach as well as digestive enzymes protect from parasite infestation. Adequate stomach acid helps protect against parasites. Regular hand washing and clean food preparation are important in disease prevention. Unfortunately, many of us need acid blockers and are not too picky about our food sources or hand-washing techniques. Just consider the all-you-can-eat buffets where you serve yourself. Do they wash those utensils between guests? How many of us take some form of acid blocker to avoid a food sensitivity or poor food combining issue. Also, because of our inability to accept the real threat of parasites, we ignore it, thus allowing it further proliferate. Parasites do nothing to help you; they are harmful. Just consider the mistletoe on the tree, a little load will generally not harm the tree; but as the load increases, the tree suffers nutritionally.

Fortunately there are many anti-parasitic herbal blends available. Parasites require a blend of herbs to destroy them, to minimize harmful effects to the body while maximizing their abilities against the parasites. Similar to tuberculosis, you do not use one medicine to destroy such

—

a tough enemy. In tuberculosis, you must take at least three separate medications to attempt to eradicate the organism and avoid resistance. Parasites also develop a resistance to herbal or pharmaceutical medicines, and you must use multiple effective remedies to remove them.

Bacteria and Viruses

Symptoms of infections from these may occur rapidly as in viral gastroenteritis and food poisoning or come on slowly, such as putrefactive bacteria.

A serious issue: if you take antibiotics for bacterial infections to the exclusion of other approaches, you will not only destroy the harmful bacteria that you are taking the antibiotic for but also destroy beneficial bacteria as well. This causes intestinal dysbiosis. Basically, sturdier toxin releasing bacteria and yeasts overgrow. It is always important to limit yeast and bacterial overgrowth with probiotics. Probiotics are the beneficial bacteria that help us process foods and form specific nutrients such as vitamin K and B. Organic yogurt can help repopulate the bowel as well but not quite as effective as quality supplements. Acidophilus, for example, is a well-known probiotic. There are many blends available.

As examples, the pathogenic bacteria *Helicobacter pylori* are common in many individuals and can damage intestinal lining quite readily if the chance is made available. Although many of us may harbor *H. pylori* without symptoms, *H. pylori* are implicated in many ulcers in the stomach in particular. Other pathogenic bacteria, such as *Escherichia coli*, may release very sickening waste products.

Some of these pathogenic organisms can be quite resistant to antibiotic therapy because this is what induced their proliferation in the first place. The antibiotics were able to destroy the bacteria we were going after but not to sterilize the entire body. The protective bacteria normal to the intestines are diminished with antibiotic use. This provides space

—

for the pathogens. Any bacteria that survive are already resistant to the antibiotic(s) used, and therefore, resistant germs proliferate. Therefore, it is prudent to avoid antibiotics when possible. Support immune function, use probiotics as necessary (especially if you must take antibiotics) and use more natural remedies such as garlic for infections.

To avoid antibiotics consider these:

- For urinary tract infections, first drink plenty of fluids. Avoid carbonated beverages that are very toxic to the urinary system. Cranberry juice is very helpful for urinary tract infections. It keeps the bacteria from clinging to the bladder wall.
- For upper respiratory infections use garlic, gargle with goldenseal and or hyssop, and even use hyssop as a nasal wash.
- For skin infections, topical antibiotics tend to be okay but also consider tea tree oil and calendula oil.
- Keeping the body as free as possible from toxic loads also allows the immune system to function at its optimum. Many herbs also stimulate immune function including mullein and Echinacea to name a few. Consider these when you are dealing with infections.

D. Ileus

Ileus is a term used to describe the condition when the bowel basically freezes in action. It says, "Better stop now, something is wrong." Ileus can be soothed and relaxed with calming antispasmodics readily, peppermint and red raspberry leaf tea make an excellent antidote; but if you are not a tea person, catnip and fennel in a children's glycerin extract may be quite relieving. Stop the pizza and other heavy foods.

Ileus also can be serious with possible pending obstruction or perforation, depending on how you react. Paralytic ileus occurs with any severe penetrating inflammation, such as with appendicitis. To help manage

—

symptoms of ileus, *do not eat*. Keep hydrated with sips of red raspberry leaf tea mixed with peppermint and nettles or maybe catnip for calming effects. I do not like the taste or smell of valerian, so valerian generally does not make it into my teas but in glycerin tinctures and powders.

Warm baths and moist compresses are helpful and soothing as well as not panicking yourself. Enemas, gently done, can be quite helpful in managing even serious ileus conditions. Enemas relieve the afterload pressure, encouraging forward flow of stool because there is no resistance. Catnip tea alone in enema form can do absolute wonders for spasm and ileus in enema form. These must be done in the care of *skillful* hands when the ileus is severe. But there is likely some surgery that could be avoided with appropriate complimentary approaches.

See a qualified physician if your symptoms are severe or involving a child and if you are at all uncomfortable about the treatments. Follow your intuition. Don't be closed to the possibilities with these approaches, but do not underestimate your intuition; and if you are not ready for this help, it probably will not help you as much anyway.

E. Headaches

Toxins released from the bowel are excreted directly, or processed by the liver and/or kidneys and later excreted. When excessive malabsorption, putrefaction, and inflammation occur, increased demand is placed in these organs of elimination. Patients ineffectively clearing toxins get headaches, nausea, and a sort of a poisoning I refer to as "brain fog."

Marshmallow root has a special role in protecting the kidneys from any insult the toxins from the bowel may cause (autointoxication). Blending marshmallow root powder into the enema tea or using sliced dried root in a tea steeped for at least fifteen minutes is helpful in preventing kidney injury from the excess toxic load.

—

Herbs helpful in promoting liver function also help in managing and eventually eliminating headaches. These include barberry, dandelion, yellow dock, yarrow, and hyssop.

For immediate relief, consider a cool compress on the head and a warm mustard footbath. Herbs for immediate relief, within thirty or forty-five minutes or so, include turmeric, meadowsweet, and willow bark for anti-inflammatory action. Catnip has a calming and muscle relaxing effect. Native Americans used bittersweet root for pain relieving qualities in low dosages. Drink plenty of fluids and of course get plenty of rest.

F. Adhesions

EFAs and fresh extra virgin olive oil are nutritive and softening for adhesions. Castor oil may help with adhesions. The external massage of castor oil into the abdomen might soften scar as well as help pain. Historically, castor oil was used as a poultice over the abdomen or liver to help dissolve calcifications and enhance immune and liver activity. With adhesions, you want to soften tissue and stimulate renewal. I believe adhesions are likely in any inflammatory conditions. Female troubles also cause adhesions, as do other illnesses such as infections, and scar tissue from abdominal surgeries is the most recognized cause. Consider topical essential oils in the care of adhesion pain, cypress oil shows promise. Rest and heal as well as you can after any surgery. Keep bowels as loose as possible and stay hydrated.

G. Pain

Pain is a signal to you that something is wrong and not functioning properly, tissues are inflamed or irritated. Do not ignore this pain.

Rest is the best thing you can do when suffering from pain.

—

Moist heat in the form of a warm wet towel or hot water bottle is very helpful in calming painful abdominal conditions.

A gentle massage with castor oil can greatly alleviate abdominal pain as well, especially when adhesions are involved. You may not know this unless testing has shown the adhesions that usually may only be seen when the abdominal cavity is opened.

Limit solid food intake as tolerated. Use juices and teas to maintain your nutrition. This will keep your nourishment up while minimizing the demands on the intestinal tract. Drink plenty of fluids.

Limit fiber if you are at risk for blockage of any kind. Flaxseed oil can be used to encourage bowel health and relieve pain when used consistently.

Enemas as previously discussed can greatly alleviate pain after a period of rest. Do these very slowly when suffering from pain and have someone around to be there if you need any help.

Herbs that have been particularly helpful with pain for me include valerian in capsule form, mullein in capsule form, and boswellia and turmeric in a quality blend or separate if that is all you can find. Gravel root and/or collinsonia are helpful in dissolving stone and adhesion formations and thus can benefit painful conditions.

Regularly include good oils in large amounts, from 1000 mg to even 10,000 mg of omega oils to protect against inflammation, one of the major causes of pain. Turmeric also has natural anti-inflammatory activity. Tart cherry syrup may help with pain as well.

If you must use pharmaceutical pain medications it is wise to avoid the stronger medicines that aggravate and cause constipation such as codeine and hydrocodone whenever possible. These medications must be prescribed by a licensed physician. Antispasmodics may help with some symptoms of cramps, but be careful as they reduce bowel motility. Try to ease up the work of and soothe the bowel in effort to reduce the need of these medications.

CHAPTER 14

Pregnancy

Reproduction is one of the most fascinating creations of God. To experience the opportunity of making a family is paramount in many people's expectations of life. Raising children is an awesome responsibility and privilege. When the mother suffers from any bowel disease, especially the more serious kinds, the disease must be maintained in its most quiescent state. Pregnancy places more demands on the mother, which in turn can greatly influence both her and her spouse's health and wellbeing.

Optimum health should be sought before any mother becomes pregnant, but this is not always the case. Unfortunately, as in many other scenarios, pregnancy may not be under the most ideal circumstances. This may be because bowel disorders can go unrecognized for years and often presents during pregnancy. In known health problems, the mother may never completely achieve that remission when pregnancy is strongly desired. In these cases, it is faith, patience, and wisdom that are necessary for the best outcome. Especially throughout pregnancy, mothers should seek to care for their bodies in a more responsible way. There is inherently much more demands on the woman's digestive system, as well as extra demands on her cardiovascular system, her eliminative organ systems (liver, skin, lungs, kidneys, and bowels), and her bloodstream.

Much success has been reported when both prospective mothers and fathers follow specific guidelines for healthier offspring and maintain their body in its most ideal health (eliminate toxins, nourish) prior to conception. In Europe, there are impressive infertility centers that have protocol to follow for eliminating toxins in and around prospective parents for at least six months prior to conception. This allows the gametes, each a half of the future child, to be in their healthiest environment and form. The groundbreaking work by Francesca Naish and Janette Roberts in their book *The Natural Way to a Better Pregnancy* is highly recommended for those seeking a better chance at a healthy pregnancy. They founded The Jocelyn Center in Sydney, Australia, a very inspirational infertility clinic dedicated to helping couples to conceive naturally and have healthy babies. Their success rate in both conception and achievement in having normal, healthy term infants is astonishing.

Bowel complaints often begin in young adults, and pregnancy, as in other stresses, provokes the impending illness. Inflammatory bowel disease often has its onset in the second and third decade of life, between ages fifteen and thirty. This disease may first manifest itself during a pregnancy as pregnancy places much demands on the body as mentioned before. Also, the symptoms can be so vague early in the disease that inflammatory bowel disease may not be recognized at the time a woman decides to have a baby. As the pregnancy advances, the disease follows. Bowel disease can put the mother at a very high risk in pregnancy, and skillful supervision is never more important than at this time.

With my pregnancies, prior to my actual awareness of my own health issues, symptoms were manifest. Uterine irritability was a regular part of the experience with three out of four of my children born preterm. As I developed understanding of nutritional health and my own situation, my babies benefitted.

—

Dietary Suggestions

It is important to have the bowel in as strong a condition as possible during pregnancy. It is even more important at this time to avoid bowel irritants such as coffee, white flour/white sugar products, cigarettes, and alcohol. Frequent small meals during the daytime with easily digestible nutritious foods are the easiest way to assimilate appropriate nutrients. It may be better to steam vegetables rather than eating them raw to improve digestibility. Soy products, carrot juice, and other super foods greatly enhance your health during pregnancy. Among some of the most important foods I recommend include blackstrap molasses, 1-2 tablespoons at least every other day or so. Blackstrap molasses contains all the organic minerals removed to produce white sugar. It may be hard to swallow at first, but after a couple days, you become accustomed to the taste. Wonderful organic calcium, iron, and potassium, as well as many trace minerals are readily absorbable and assimilable. This means the minerals go straight to nervous, bone, and other tissues efficiently. Your offspring get more available nutrients for tissues including nerve and bone, and your own bone density improves.

Juices

Carrot juice, as fresh as possible, was extremely helpful in providing nutrition to my baby and me, being easily digested and very nourishing. I recommend using organic carrots to minimize exposures to pesticides, but if unavailable, buy regular grocery store type carrots and wash extremely well. Carrot juice is helpful to maintain blood sugar levels, and making a pitcher to have on hand is worthwhile to encourage drinking more frequently. Fresh juice only keeps a day, so finish what you make. Also, in the literature, there is valid concern that bruising and rotting of fruits and vegetables can damage intestinal lining itself from toxic byproducts in the decomposing foods. Be careful about the quality and condition of the produce you use.

Vegetable and fruit juices can be a worthwhile investment toward a healthy pregnancy. Juiced vegetables and fruits are easier to digest and absorb. Carrot juice is sweet and should be used in small portions such as 1 or 2 ounces. Other vegetables are not so sweet and can be used to dilute the carrots. Celery contains silica as well as organic calcium, and although can be stringy to juice, is wonderful to mix with carrot juice for a healthy beverage. Beetroots are very nutritional but should only be used sparingly or with caution, as they can cause some internal cleansing, which may cause toxins to release into the bloodstream therefore exposing the fetus with previously stored-away toxins. Beets are better utilized in cleansing practices prior to conception. Apples can be easily juiced including its stem, seeds, and all. It is preferred not to mix fruit juices with vegetable juices, although apple and carrot combine well. There is concern over the pesticides used in fruits such as apples, and indeed commercial apple juice is at risk. Apples should be organic or at least washed thoroughly. Small amounts of parsley may also blend nicely with carrots, adding some bitterness as well as more organic calcium, minerals, and silica. Silica is important to the development of strong bones and various forms of connective tissue, working adjunctively with calcium. Remember you do not have to juice these foods for benefit, just concentrated benefit.

Many juices are available commercially. Grape is particularly gentle and slightly cleansing. Apple juice can be cooling to some and, therefore, should often be diluted with pure water. Orange juice can be hard to tolerate by some but does aid in the absorption and utilization of medicines and herbs and rapidly improves blood sugar levels. Grapefruit juice is healthful, although there are precautions in drinking grapefruit juice with medications as the medications are so rapidly absorbed. This can cause the pharmaceutical medications to act much stronger and potentially could have dangerous consequences. Cranberry juice, somewhat bitter, has added

–

benefits of protecting against bladder infections so prevalent in pregnant women. All juices should be of the best quality you can afford.

Other Nutritious Foods

As previously discussed, the bitter taste is very beneficial to digestion, and mixed green salads including watercress, sorrel, dandelion, and dark green lettuces chewed well can wonderfully nourish the mother and infant. Other super foods include sprouts of various grains, such as wheat grass and barley. These sprouts can be added to your juice as well as added to salads and sandwiches with much benefit.

There is such a variety of foods that can greatly benefit the mother and baby. Salads, as well as all raw vegetables, should be thoroughly chewed, especially when digestion is impaired in any way. As mentioned earlier, fruits should not only be chewed well but also eaten separately from proteins (other than possibly soy, which does not get so adversely impacted in digestion when combined with fruit; soy is more digestible and alkaline.) Also, vegetables are more digestible steamed and, thus, may benefit more as the nutrients, even though a small amount may be lost to the vapor, will be more available.

Unsaturated fresh oils such as wheat germ oil and olive oil, as well as essential fatty acids, are very beneficial to the mother and baby during pregnancy and beyond. Essential fatty acid intake should be adequate for not only the developing baby but also for nourishing nervous health and keeping inflammation in check. Flax seed oil, borage seed oil, and evening primrose seed oil are all healthy safe important supplements in pregnancy. Avocadoes are especially helpful in providing healthy fats during pregnancy.

Grape seed oil is not recommended because of some potentially toxic constituents. During this more sensitive time avoid "proinflammatory"

—

fats, such as those from red meat (saturated) and margarine (artificially saturated).

Other nutritious foods for pregnancy include kelp as a seasoning, slowly cooked beans, and wholesome vegetables. All these can be combined into a very nourishing soup. Also, small fish from clean water sources is exceptionally healthy for the pregnant mother and unborn child.

Herbs

Many herbal teas can benefit both mother and baby. Again, my favorite red raspberry leaf tea is safe and wonderfully nutritive. Red raspberry leaves have an extremely long history of use in pregnancy, beneficial in strengthening the reproductive organs as well as alleviating symptoms of morning sickness, the nausea in pregnancy that may occur any time but most commonly during the morning of the first trimester when the body is adjusting to the hormonal shifts. Although theoretically, some herbals suggest avoiding red raspberry tea in early pregnancy from a suspected higher risk of miscarriage from stimulation of the uterus, this assumption has not borne out. As a word of caution though, it may be advisable to limit the tea use in the first trimester to a few cups a day. Red raspberry leaves do help make the birthing process more efficient, but this does not mean this tea stimulates labor. The tea seems to nourish and tonify the pelvic structures, therefore making childbirth more efficient and the perineum more elastic, not directly stimulating the uterus as proposed in some literature. Many gifted, experienced herbalists highly endorse the use of red raspberry leaf tea in pregnancy, including me. Other wonderful teas in pregnancy include stinging nettle (does not have irritant properties when put in tea form or cooked), chamomile and catnip.

Licorice is especially useful to both maintain control of and decrease the requirements of prednisone for inflammation but should be used with caution because of its ability to raise blood pressure and its estrogenic and mineralocorticoid (changes the balance of water and minerals) activities. It is significantly safer than prednisone and very effective at controlling inflammation when from a good source but should be used in the lowest effective doses, such as one-two capsules a day or every other day. Severe inflammatory bowel disease is likely more harmful in pregnancy than the daily small doses of licorice necessary to limit the disease activity. Licorice cannot always control the disease alone though; add mullein and slippery elm to your regimen as well as gentle enemas, dietary guidelines, and plenty of rest all in an effort to contribute to a healthy pregnancy and baby. Bleeding from the bowel at this time can greatly affect the health of the mother and baby by increasing the risk for anemia already present in pregnancy. Shepherd's purse in small doses may stop gastrointestinal bleeding but be aware that it may thicken blood as well as stimulate uterine contractions. Shepherds purse has been used regularly by skillful midwives to control uterine hemorrhage. There are some reports this herb is additive in effect due to presence of oxytocin, a uterine contraction stimulant, thus potentially stimulating early labor or miscarriage; but this is not seen at all in the small doses effective in managing active bleeding. Used in low doses for bleeding episodes and not for prevention, shepherds purse is safe for most.

A Final Note

Please take active responsibility of your health especially this time in order to have the healthiest baby and pregnancy possible, so seek the advice of gifted, skillful, knowledgeable healers, both conventional and alternative. A mother has the real responsibility in having a healthy baby not the physician at hand. They must work together. Too many people give the responsibility of maintaining their health to physicians when the real responsibility lies within the patient.

—

CHAPTER 15

Healing Whole Foods

For rapidly growing children as well as adults, it is important to provide the best nutrition you can. Sometimes this is not easy with children having such a predisposition for sweets and breads. This is fast energy for them but ultimately depleting. Certain foods can help you in restoring mineral, vitamin, and other nutritional status for improved health and resistance to disease. These foods tend to be highly concentrated sources of nutrients, so it does not take a lot for most children. A few I find very useful are listed below.

Blackstrap molasses (organic)

This byproduct of the processing of white sugar is loaded with nutrients especially valuable minerals such as calcium and organic potassium. Small teaspoonfuls every other day can have dramatic results. Larger and older children can have more. I do not find this supplement particularly tasty but worth the medicine. Look for better nervous development and bone mass for starters.

Royal bee jelly

This is the substance from worker bees that converts a larvae into a new queen bee. A queen bee lives over 20 times longer than the others. This is a well-known complete nutrition source and can be especially useful for growing children.

Whole food concentrates

There are various products available that concentrate whole vegetables and fruits in gummy bear-type supplements and tablet forms. Hero has Yummi Bears. These are worth the expense, especially if you have finicky eaters.

Wheat germ oil

You might consider supplementing your children with a small teaspoon of this oil, fresh, for super vitamin E. This oil can also be rubbed into the skin. Consider the risk of wheat allergy though when using this oil.

Natural sweeteners and Honey

Honey is a fascinating sweetener with antibacterial and healing properties. There was concern about infants getting botulism from poorly stored honey though, so it is recommended to avoid for the infant until the age of one year. This theoretical risk is not worth taking. With much restorative, nutritive, and antibacterial properties, the food can be very useful in multiple ways from treating a sore throat to coating over an open wound.

—

Natural sweeteners such as maple syrup and stevia leaf have nutritional value.

Spirulina/ Blue-green algae/ Kelp/ Chlorella

These dark green usually amino acid-rich foods contain minerals, alginate, chlorophyll, and numerous other substances. Get these supplements from quality sources. It is hard to get a child to take these, as they are usually available in capsule or tablet form, but try adding a little kelp to "salt" your soup and other possible meals.

Many chlorophyll rich foods such as dark colored vegetables and fruits can be eaten in abundance. Take advantage of the healthful foods available. Juicing can concentrate the nutrients. Be sure to wash the produce well and have ample supply available. Eat your daily vegetables.

Celery

Learn to love celery. The silica and minerals found in it cannot be matched, and celery is very cleansing as well. Teeth, bone, and collagen everywhere, plus all that depend on calcium can be nourished with celery.

Carrots

Carrots do have many valuable organic minerals, but what comes to mind most is the valuable and natural vitamin A in the form of beta-carotene that supports healing and proper growth.

Beets

Beets are very cleansing so use with care in more delicate or toxic individuals. Beets, with their dark purple color, are an ultimate blood builder as well as cleanser. Beets help liver function. Generally, young children will not like the taste of beets, but you can include some of the root in your juices, mixed with carrot juice for an extremely nourishing drink.

Berries and Cherries

These fruits are loaded in nutrients valuable for long-term health. Most individuals enjoy these fruits but they must be readily available. Blueberries are a wonderful support to not only the blood vessels but the nervous system as well. Cherries are especially nutritious as well as soothing and aid in lung function as well as arthritis. Black cherries show promise in gout as well as other arthritis complaints.

Olive oil

I consider this a super food. Cook often with this oil. Extra virgin oil is the most pure form. Olive oil contains an abundance of polyunsaturated and monounsaturated oils, essential to nerve and all membrane development. If you have a very ill child who cannot eat, consider a nice warm olive oil massage to encourage some type of nutrition support. You will be impressed. Olive oil is more stable in heat than other polyunsaturated oils, but still, users should smell and taste for any rancidity. Rancid oil is extremely harmful especially with repeated use.

–

Oats

Oats are extremely nourishing, very calming, and supportive especially to nervous tissue. Encourage your child to eat oatmeal regularly, as wholesome and fresh as possible. Don't destroy the benefit by adding a large amount of sugar but consider maple syrup, honey, and/or a few berries instead as a sweetener.

Dark leafy green lettuce

Include mixed green salads in your diet, especially the dark leaf types. These salad greens are loaded with valuable minerals as well as the indispensable chlorophyll. Chlorophyll provides at least building blocks for blood and oxygenation.

Broccoli

Broccoli can be quite nutritious steamed. There is some concern about the calcium oxalates; these may be difficult to process in some people. But in modest usage, broccoli is already loaded with nutrients.

When you are using fresh produce, be sure to wash it well to avoid and minimize any contamination.

Soy

Soy foods might be appreciated and utilized. Soy is relatively cheap on resources as well as monetarily in the grocery store. Soy is a great healer. Soy can be sensitizing to some but still many can benefit from soy's proteins and oils as well as other factors. Soy has a perfect amino acid protein balance and is alkalinizing.

Nuts and Seeds

Fresh peanuts are wholesome, especially when you buy organic and the freshest available. Commercial peanut butter may be wholesome but may be contaminated with aflatoxin, so buy premium brands. Peanuts, although well rounded in proteins, are deficient in many beneficial fatty acids as compared to other nuts and seeds. Seeds such as sunflower have good oils and proteins. Almonds are another consideration. There are indeed a variety of nuts that offer unique valuable balances of nutrients with their essential fatty acid content. Walnuts and pine nuts are additionally anti-parasitic, Nut milks and butters may be a better choice for some as digestion problems can be exacerbated by undigested fragments.

Organic

Organic foods are grown under different environmental conditions than regular produce. The land must be rotated; the soil must be rich in natural compost nutrients. Kelp is very helpful in an organic garden for nutritionally restoring depleted soils that have not been cared for. Buying organic generally means no chemical fertilizers or pesticides have been used, making the produce safer.

Genetically modified foods (GMO)

These can possibly be organic, but they have been manipulated in their genetic code. For example, fish flounder DNA (fragments of the genetic code) might be inserted into corn, allowing corn to become more cold resistant. There is unfortunately much genetic manipulation in our food supply. Soy beans, corn, and other grains, should be watched for genetic modification. This improves the crop yield with undernourished soils; the plants do not have to be as hardy on their own. This manipulation may not produce more nourishing produce, ultimately allowing for illness. Strong, healthy plants grown in natural environments have been shown to be more nourishing.

Additives and artificial flavors and colors

Another addition too much of our commercial food, these substances are used to extend the shelf life and improve the color or flavor for desirability. Unfortunately, these substances can be very damaging for some individuals, especially children, who tend to consume more of these type of foods.

Being realistic, we all may eat candy or cupcakes, what I am really trying to reinforce is moderation. It was very enlightening when I found some leftover cupcakes from four or more months ago in a cabinet that I had forgotten about. They looked fresh, probably did not feel that way, but the color of the frosting was as brilliant as ever and there was no mold in sight. I threw them out immediately lest my children find them and think I had bought them recently. Not even mold grow on these things.

Another thing to consider, those tiny insects that invade your grains and waste a lot of money in damaged food; they won't go near granulated sugar.

With all the depression, anxiety, and attention problems in our country, it is wise to consider reading labels more regularly for possible harmful substances. You want foods in the most natural state as possible, with as little chemical intervention as available. Also, many cancers and unusual immune-type diseases may be improved with a cleaner diet and lifestyle. Remember, we need to restore and maintain our physical health as a priority; what we eat and are exposed to do affect our capabilities, stamina, and overall health.

Thermal properties of foods

Depending on the temperature of the food as well as the heating effect from spices, certain foods are tolerated better by certain individuals. To clarify, if you have a weak child or a sensitive individual, it is unwise to give them a large amount of raw foods to ingest. Their body must not only undergo more work in digestive processes but must use energy to warm foods to body temperature. On the other hand, if you have an overheated individual, it may be wise to encourage cooler fluids to aid in cooling the body, unless the person is acute. Then you must consider neutral temperatures to allow the body to gradually cool down safely. Individuals with type O blood tend to be more robust and can tolerate cooler foods. They have excessive heat often from a meat diet as well as from predisposition. More delicate individuals may not tolerate cold foods and beverages as well, so it is important to individualize.

Be gentle with your children when they are in a delicate condition; give them warmer foods and plenty of fluids. Do not use too much stimulating or hot foods or herbs. Find the foods that are the most nutritious as well as easily digestible. This can be a problem with children though, as some can be quite finicky when ill. In this case, encourage much nutritious herbal teas adequately sweetened to improve the child's energy. Carrot juice in this case might be allowed to warm to room temperature or just below it rather than stay chilled (although must always be fresh). Vegetable soup is appropriate for most.

—

Foods are inherently warming, cooling, or neutral. For example, jalapeno peppers are definitely warming. In weakened individuals, some foods such as these are too hot for the time being. As foundation is strengthened more stimulating and heating herbals can help. There is a balance to the thermal properties that is more routinely approached in Chinese medicine.

Warming foods include onions, garlic (very warming), squash, spelt, cherries, oats, asparagus, artichoke, and potatoes. Parsley is slightly warming.

Cooling foods could include wheat, apples, pears, oranges, strawberries, bananas, eggplant, spinach, sweet potato, avocado, and lettuce. This is why apple juice is potentially depleting even if you dilute the sugar content.

Neutral foods include rice, rye, carrots, beets, potatoes, plums, apricots, figs, grapes, pineapples, raspberries, and papaya.

Consider not only the taste sensation but also the temperature quality of the everyday foods you ingest and feed your children. To encourage their vitality, choose for them the most appropriate foods. Sometimes, choose raw foods to cool down a child, other times steam the same foods to keep the child warm or neutral. In the summer, you eat watermelon, in the winter, you eat potatoes. As you learn to avoid synthetic foods, white sugar, and white flour, you begin to be drawn more toward healthful foods. This is a long process though in many cases, as our tastebuds have become so confused.

Cooking can be valuable in improving digestibility as well as destroying parasites and other organisms to protect the delicate intestinal lining in susceptible individuals.

Molds

I am quite concerned about the increasing mold in our foods and atmosphere. Some molds are quite harmless and even useful, such as usnea and chlorella. But certain molds that most determine the shelf life of foods produce toxic substances. Most notorious among these are aflatoxin and ergot. These types of molds are very damaging when one is exposed to them, especially chronically. There is a study available demonstrating patients may be more susceptible to mental illness because of these food exposures. The problem is not only with the molds themselves but also in the chemicals used to prevent the growth. Both are not harmless; not only must you watch out for the preservatives used to lengthen shelf life, but you also must stay aware of the time foods have remained on your own shelves, especially organic foods. This also implies purchasing from reputable sources; consider both brand name and store.

Aflatoxin harbors ergotlike substances with possible effects of hallucinations and other impaired-thinking processes. Aflatoxin is from contaminated nuts that have been improperly dried. Ergot is from improperly dried wheat and other grain products. Aflatoxin and ergot are toxins created from the mold contaminant. Consider mold exposure if there are any mental issues, especially any with delusional thinking. The Salem witch hunts were the result of ergot, very similar to an LSD reaction. These women, because they alone did not quite understand what they were dealing with, may have been quite frightened with early symptoms of ergot poisoning with stale grains.

Aflatoxin causes more of a headache-type reaction that has more long-term consequences.

Aflatoxin can be in moldy produce as well as nuts.

Be sure to trim and wash your produce well, and eat your bread-type foods as fresh as possible. Don't even let the birds eat moldy bread.

Also, remember to consider rancidity as a factor in preventing health problems and maintaining a healthful fatty acid status and function.

CHAPTER 16

Nutritional Supplements

Certain supplements may be particularly beneficial for patients with bowel disorders. The supplements listed below I have used with significant responses and minimal, if no, side effects. These are readily available at health food stores and should be of fresh, high quality. Certain supplements, such as essential fatty acid oils and acidophilus, must be refrigerated to preserve their shelf life. I would like to present a brief description of some of my favorite supplements with regard to bowel disease.

1. **Acidophilus Culture**—It is best to refrigerate this substance as previously mentioned. There are a variety of beneficial bacteria, lactobacillus and other species, that are necessary to support health. They manufacture certain vitamins, for example, various B vitamins, and are an especially important source of vitamin B12. These bacteria are considered protective to the human body, blocking the ability of more pathogenic organisms to colonize the bowel. Acidophilus and related bacterial species as well as certain yeasts also play an important role in breaking down undigested

fermenting foods. There are a variety of beneficial bacteria, and it is best to get supplements that contain different species not just one strain. It is especially necessary for patients to supplement with quality acidophilus preparations when they take antibiotics. In general, I frequently recommend yogurt as a healthy source of beneficial flora although the dairy is so mucus thickening. Yogurt is certainly nourishing and easy to digest, and in my opinion its benefits often outweigh its risks. For example, in patients treated for respiratory complaints, the dairy in yogurt may thwart efforts at a healthy recovery slightly; but with adequate fluids, they still get well and rarely ever get yeast or gastrointestinal complications. If you are severely depleted though and are having to take antibiotics, yogurt is advised as well as adequately nourishing fluids.

2. **Adrenal Gland**—This is an animal product which may be very useful in building up a deficient individual. Adrenal fatigue is a relatively common problem, affecting most of us when we are under chronic stress, as in any chronic disease situation. Be sure to buy from a reputable source, organic and free-range animals. Use small amounts, one-two capsules a day. I tend to suggest minimizing use of animal glandular. Life begets life, and glandular do not seem to carry the life giving qualities I prefer.

3. **Apple Cider Vinegar**—I have found this food to be stimulating and regulating to the digestive system as well as detoxifying. Use organic non-filtered varieties. Put 3 tablespoons in a glass or cup of warm water and sweeten with honey and lemon as desired. Take in the morning a half hour or so before breakfast for significant tonic effects.

4. **Alpha-lipoic Acid** (thioctic acid)—This supplement is very beneficial to patients with liver disease as well as neuropathies by protecting cells and stimulating regeneration. The supplement functions as a coenzyme and antioxidant, especially protecting the

—

liver. By stimulating nerve tissue regeneration, the supplement has shown consistent reversal of liver disease as well as neuropathies of various causes. This supplement is easily absorbed, interacting with other antioxidants to scavenge free radicals. The supplement is considered preventive against cancer. Lipoic acid also enhances oxygenation of tissues in addition to reducing lactic acid levels, thus improving energy levels. The substance is found in abundance in potatoes and other mitochondria rich foods.

Donnie Yance, a respected, if not revered, herbal healer dedicated to cancer victims, recommends alpha-lipoic acid highly for any type of liver disease or dysfunction.

5. **Bee Pollen**—Extremely nourishing, bee pollen is said to bring on the "spring bloom" in horses. There are many trace minerals and substances that greatly benefit vitality. Potentially, local bee honey is protective against allergic symptoms. Very well tolerated, no known side effects. It is best to refrigerate this substance to improve the shelf life.

6. **Bentonite Clay**—This substance is especially absorptive, extracting various substances, especially toxins, from the digestive tract when ingested. You should take clay with plenty of fluids; and it is best to take this clay with psyllium, which will be discussed later. Psyllium improves the consistency of the clay. Caution is warranted with psyllium husks though, as these can be very irritating and allergenic. There is also some concern I have with the possibility of aluminum in clay; but because the clay is so absorbent, this aluminum should not be left behind in your body. This clay can be very useful in alleviating symptoms of gastritis or heartburn because of its immediate effects. Clay can also be helpful in absorbing toxins created further down in the colon, the process referred to as autointoxication. This effect is not as rapidly noticed, but over time, there are consistent beneficial results. I

would recommend if you want to try this supplement to take the clay for three-four days in a row, then stop to allow your body to rest from the detoxification, especially if you have lower bowel disease. Also, be sure to drink plenty of pure water when you use clay as a supplement.

7. **Black Cherry Syrup**—This tasty sweetener is loaded with organic minerals. Also, it is very soothing especially to the respiratory system. I periodically give my children with bowel disorders black cherry syrup to supplement their mineral status, and I get very little to no resistance from them. This food is also very easy on the stomach. I have found cherry syrup useful for coughs as well as gout, and other painful arthritis complaints.

8. **Blackstrap molasses**—This is the byproduct of sugar cane in the processing of sugar, thus many elemental minerals are readily available to the body. This food is extremely useful for deficient persons. The minerals especially support the skeletal and nervous system, and all tissues are nourished as well. I recommend getting organic blackstrap molasses. Beware that not all molasses is blackstrap molasses and read your labels. Molasses in general grocery stores is often "flavored" molasses. Blackstrap, with all of the minerals it contains, heals and builds bones and other tissues. Blackstrap molasses is especially useful in osteoporosis and injuries, as well as in childhood growth.

9. **Butyrate**—Found in butter and in smaller amounts in cottage cheese, yogurt, and other dairy foods, butyrate is also available as a supplement. Butyrate is protective to the intestinal lining and strongly associated with protection against colon cancer. Butyrate is a fuel for beneficial bacteria.

10. **Coenzyme Q10**—this substance is important for metabolism and oxygenation of tissues, with significant antioxidant protection. The supplement has been proven to be extremely beneficial in

heart disease as well as being protective for all the cells in the body. A good dose in most patients would be 50 milligrams daily, although doses as high as 100 milligrams would significantly benefit most patients. Higher doses help muscle pain and fatigue. The supplement is expensive but well worth the investment if you have any kind of heart disease at all, especially when you have a serious heart disease. The supplement is safe. I have found report of rare palpitations with coenzyme q10 and have seen possibly two episodes. I start patients low, from 30-100 mg daily. If they have no problem we can bring the dose up, and in some 400 mg twice a day truly benefits their muscular pains and fatigue. Their skin notably looks healthier. I have found great benefit with CoQ10. It can be costly, but I do not think you need the most expensive formula for benefit. There are often sales, and if you feel better, you might find the expense worth it.

11. **Colloidal silver**, for infections. This supplement is not for prolonged periods of time.

12. **Colostrum**—The first milk of cows, colostrum is loaded with immune factors, building blocks, and other substances. Consider using after you have been cleansing a while to sort of 'reset' the immune system. This is not necessarily a long-term treatment, but a week or two of daily doses of colostrum should be considered. Potentially you would get milk allergy symptoms as a possible side effect to this supplement, but it tends to be well tolerated by many to build up a deficient person.

13. **Essential fatty acids**—These vital nutrients are sorely deficient in many individuals, and as previously mentioned earlier in my book, these must be supplemented. You cannot take too much of these. They are available in many different oils grouped here. These primarily include the oils made from flaxseed, black currant seed, evening primrose seed, borage seed, and fish. Be careful with fish

liver oil. This oil contains large quantities of vitamin D and A, which could be harmful if taken in large doses. The benefit of the fish liver oil is the already formed prostaglandins, docasohexanoic acid (DHA), and eicasopentanoic acid (EPA), which are available to tissues such as nervous tissue. The other oils must be transformed in the liver to these vital fatty acids among other vital fatty acid products. If the liver is poorly functioning, it may not be capable of providing adequate amounts of these substances, causing deficiency and poor vitality. In patients with healthy livers, flaxseed oil is a very good source of the precursors to EPA and DHA. Fatty acids are necessary for every cell membrane in the body, and when they are deficient, fluidity of cellular structures is lost among other problems. Hardening arteries and poor skin are just some of the results. Supplementation with essential fatty acids is especially necessary to check inflammation in a healthy, natural way. These must be fresh. Never use omega oils that smell bad. Rancid oils are harmful. Symptoms of rancid oils include burping and nausea.

14. **Fructo-oligosaccharides (FOS)**—This supplement is a valuable source of nutrition for beneficial bacteria. The supplement encourages beneficial bacteria to proliferate and adequately colonize the intestinal tract, promoting restoration of the balance necessary for health. FOS molecules are smaller sugar-type starches nutritive for friendly bacteria. This supplement goes well with supplementation of acidophilus and related beneficial bacteria.

15. **Glutamine**—An important amino acid widely available. This particular amino is an important food source to the intestinal lining, and supplementation may be very beneficial for those suffering with bowel disease, especially inflammations where cell turnover and energy use is high. An opened capsule of glutamine may be useful in hypoglycemia when placed under the tongue; the protein is small enough to be absorbed in this way efficiently.

—

16. **Glycine**—a short amino acid is an important building block for intestinal cells and cells in the nervous system. Can be used in very weakened bowels, especially with glutamate.

17. **Methylsulfonylmethane (MSM)**—This substance is manufactured and is similar to dimethylsulfoxide (DMSO) without the odor. The supplement is extremely anti-inflammatory and provides vital sulfur for tissues such as the liver cells to improve detoxification mechanisms. I find this supplement especially beneficial to those with bowel inflammation as well as peripheral inflammations such as arthralgia and arthritis. Take two-ten grams a day for significant benefit, lesser in a child depending on weight.

18. **N-acetyl-glucosamine**—This is intestinal-lining food and is very helpful in helping support healing tissues of the lining. Can be used daily safely.

19. **Psyllium**—This is an excellent fiber source taken with plenty of water. The fiber has potential use in absorbing toxins created in the bowel as well as to establish bowel regularity. Unfortunately, this particular fiber has had an increased recognition of allergic reactions, possibly related to its irritant properties or to more frequent usage. If you have active inflammation and raw tissues, you may want to use slippery elm instead. Psyllium seed can be somewhat better tolerated by soaking the whole seed for several hours and crushed to eat as gruel.

20. **Royal Bee Jelly**—Similar as bee pollen, nutritionally, but more ring structures for hormone precursors. This is what the Queen bee ingests.

21. **Thymus gland**—Consider this supplement for patients with severe immune system deregulation under expertise advice. Use small amounts from a reputable source for 3 or more months after having corrected as much with the immune exposures and issues. There are mixed philosophies on organ supplementation, and I am cautious about routine use of this. It may be considered in severe situations.

—

CHAPTER 17

Favorite Herbal Medicines

This is list somewhat in two orders, the most necessary to know now, and alphabetical.

1. Catnip leaves (*Nepeta cataria*). These leaves grow readily throughout much of the United States and should be in every home garden. They brew into a wonderful, relaxing, slightly cleansing tea with much nutritive value. Catnip leaves are also at the forefront as an herbal "tea" for enema use. The action is mild, consistent, stops spasms, and gently cleanses away toxic matter. Catnip is extremely safe and can be used in teas throughout pregnancy and by young children. In fact, many glycerin tincture glands are available with catnip and usually blended with fennel for colic and gas pain in children. This same formula would be very useful in adults as well. Catnip leaves combine well with other teas such as red raspberry leaves.

2. Red raspberry leaves (*Rubus strigosus*). Full of minerals, bioflavanoids, and antioxidants, this herb supports elasticity. There are astringent properties that allow the tea to assist in clearing sinuses and lungs.

Red raspberry leaves are gently cleansing and especially nourishing. I highly recommend this tea in mid to late pregnancy and for the use of children and adults. Red raspberry leaf tea makes a good base tea for all other blends. The red raspberry leaves should be young and dried properly if not used fresh. If you do not like the taste of red raspberry leaf tea, try another brand. I have found they vary much in regard to quality. You might grow and harvest your own. This plant grows quite readily if you find the correct species for your local area. A garden in itself is especially therapeutic, and this plant generally does not take so much room.

There are warnings about using red raspberry during the first trimester of a pregnancy, and it is prudent to minimize use at this time. Small amounts would be safe. Red raspberry helps nausea but peppermint tea may be a better choice in early pregnancy. Red raspberry leaf tea indeed is a pregnant woman's tea, but use later in pregnancy more freely. Children and all adults would benefit much from the healing powers available in this simple plant.

3. Anise seed (*Pimpinella anisum*) Anise tastes quite sweet and is very restorative for bowel tissues. The seeds volatile oils are especially relaxing and help to relieve nausea, gas discomfort and spasms. The delicate oils can be easily lost to vapor when preparing a tea with the seeds; these should be crushed and prepared in a tea simmered with the lid in place. Anise is also available in glycerin tinctures. The seeds are extremely safe and can be taken freely as a tea. If you grow anise, try eating a bite from the flowering tops.

4. Peppermint leaves (*Mentha pipperita*) This herb grows so freely it is obvious everyone should have it. The plant smells wonderful and has the power to relax the most spastic bowel. The herb is most easily used in a tea blend and adds flavor. The oil is the most medicinal component, with tonic qualities. The leaves should be gently dried for tea, and the tea should not be left in too hot

—

conditions. As is with many herbs with delicate volatile oils, the oils can evaporate while the tea is brewing if the lid of the pan is not in place. Oils vaporize readily. Use low heat and keep lidded.

Although natural peppermint is very helpful for stomach upset, peppermint is also available in enteric-coated capsules, capsules that do not dissolve in the stomach but in the intestine. This allows the medicine to go directly to the irritation and spasm and is quite useful for any indigestion and nausea. In restauraunts, the after dinner mints are there for a reason, although you should wait at least a half hour or more so you do not impair digestion (food combining principles.) The original after dinner mints were mints. Peppermint is also an extremely safe plant.

5. Turmeric root (*Curcuma longa*). This powerful Eastern herb is so very well known in other parts of the world and is widely available. The plant root, or rhizome as it is actually termed, is extremely medicinal. The anti-inflammatory effects are profound, especially within the gastrointestinal system. The root is known to inhibit colon cancer, is anti-parasitic, and should be on every shelf of those with bowel inflammation in particular but also for inflammation in other areas as well. Even though the herb is poorly absorbed from the bowel, the benefit to joint pains as well as abdominal pain is profound, suggesting the plant may be working by healing "leaky bowel," that lining damage which allows immune complexes to escape into the blood to accumulate in susceptible tissues. Turmeric is a maintenance medicine for many, it helps keep all inflammation at bay. You might combine with boswellia for additive benefits to joint pain.

Turmeric has the ability to thin the blood so monitor for any bleeding. The healing to the intestines may ultimately stop the bleeding cause. If you are bleeding from your intestines, do not assume it is only turmeric and have this evaluated.

—

6. Boswellia (*Boswellia serrata*). This anti-inflammatory seems to get absorbed better than turmeric and has additive effects. Boswellia is fortunately becoming more available; another Eastern herb that has found ample purpose here.

   Generally with boswellia, you do not notice an effect until days or maybe even a week or two before starting the supplement. But often when the supplement finally is used regularly, the benefit is unmistakable. The herb is available readily in capsule form, and as previously mentioned, should be used with turmeric for additive benefit; these herbs though are not cheap.

   Boswellia also potentially increases the risk of bleeding by virtue of the anti-inflammatory effects.

7. Mullein leaves and flowers (*Verbascum thapsus*). This plant is an absolute miracle plant. Historically thought of as a "glandular," mullein is irreplaceable in my own regimen, which I keep as simple as possible. Mullein seems to have restored bowel function like no other herb, and if you think about it, the digestive tract is full of glands. Mullen is incredibly useful for lung afflictions. Mullen greatly supports lung function and structure, it does not dilate the lungs, rather it supports the cells themselves. People have without a doubt learned the value of mullein.

   I take the herb leaves and flowering tops in capsule form every day. Not that the herb could have replaced other approaches, but it certainly has been one of the main contributors to my health.

   Mullein is extremely safe, and there are no known problems from taking this plant. Historically, the plant was used for baby diapers because the leaves are very large and soft. Boy scouts have been taught it is nature's tissue paper.

8. Hawthorn berry leaves and flowers (*Cratageus oxyacantha*). Although traditionally not an intestinal herb, this herb deserves honorable mention. The plant tastes very well in tea form, but also

—

can be purchased in capsules and concentrated extracts (Gaia). The plant is best known for its healing effects on the heart, but this effect expands to include all blood vessels. The herb has been proven to strengthen the heart; heart failure symptoms have been documented showing proof other than "field experience." The berries, leaves, and flowers nourish the inner lining of the heart and vessels, supporting their action and strength. Hawthorn berry needs to be more aggressively used and studied; indeed, I believe it has great possibilities not only in healing heart and vessel disease but also in aiding healing in any other tissues by supporting the blood supply.

Hawthorn berry has much benefit to every age group. There are reports of this herb helping attention deficit syndrome; and based on Chinese medicine, the ties to the heart and mind certainly could be involved in the benefit here. Hawthorn is a relaxing herb as well as heart tonic. Hawthorn berry is quite safe, and may allow the tapering of other more toxic heart medications with continued use. If you are on heart medications, let your doctor know you want to use hawthorn then gently taper the other medications, as you no longer need them. As a matter of fact, all berries are extremely heart beneficial as well as the remainder of the circulatory system.

9. Burdock (*Arctium lappa*). This root is a powerful ally in blood cleansing. The weed is widely available and easily cultivated. The tea does not taste well, but by combining this herb with peppermint and red raspberry, you would not notice.

The root is extremely nutritive, containing inulin; a most powerful healing nutritive well tolerated by diabetics because the type of sugar is different, all natural, easily assimilated, and not insulin requiring or provoking. The root is used as food in other countries, called "gobo." You may consider growing this plant, and after thorough washing and scrubbing, cooking it as a vegetable for the evening meal. The health benefit would be astonishing.

10. Barberry (*Berberis officinale*). Barberry root is the plant Dr. Christopher routinely used to help people who could not eat. The herb has powerful effects on the liver, and not only supports liver activity but also gallbladder function. Barberry is widely available, and a ready substitute with extremely similar properties would be Oregon grape (*Mahonia repens*) also widely available. This plant is a stronger purifier. The plant is very safe in itself but by nature of the cleansing action toxins will be released. When toxins reach the blood stream the body feels it. This is especially risky during pregnancy as all the blood feeds the baby. Indeed keep any cleansing to a minimum while pregnant. Therefore, barberry should not be used during pregnancy unless the symptoms of nausea are severe, and then only used in small amounts.

11. Aloe vera (*Aloe vera*). The magical aloe vera is one of the most well-known contemporary herbs of today. The inner leaf gel contains allantoin, a known cell proliferant, as well as other nutritive substances. Aloe speeds healing wherever it is used and is tolerated well taken orally as well as is used on the skin. On the skin, the most common use is for burns, but other wounds benefit just as well. When taken orally, aloe does have some laxative properties and does best when taken with other herbs; otherwise, the laxative potential can be quite powerful. The juice is anti-inflammatory and has antibiotic properties. The juice is also thought to help digestive enzymes.

12. Astragalus (*Astragalus membranaceus*). This plant is a very important and effective immune modulator and is safe for all kinds of immune deficiencies as well as overactive conditions. Used for thousands of years in China, the plant has a tremendous safety record. The constituents improve immune function by various

—

well-researched mechanisms. Astragalus is also known as a blood builder and especially increases white blood cell activity.

13. Licorice root (*Glycyrrhiza glabra*). This powerful plant has many medicinal contents including glycyrrhizin, thought to be the most active compound. All the constituents though work together to make the medicinal activity of this extremely valuable herb. This plant is anti-allergenic, anti-inflammatory, and anti-arthritic. The root also has gentle laxative effects and is very healing to the bowel lining. The root also improves lung function and is healing for asthmatic conditions as well.

There is valid concern that licorice may cause similar side effects as the pharmaceutical drug cortisone; many of the powerful components mimic this powerful hormone. I have found this plant can replace the use of prednisone/cortisone type medications by supporting the adrenal function as opposed to substituting for it.

In any event, watch for increased blood pressure and fluid retention when using this plant. A few capsules in the morning certainly would not harm most and instead benefit most of us with bowel or inflammatory disorders and is much safer than pharmaceutical cortisone preparations; but dosing higher than this increases the risk for side effects mentioned above. Sometimes though, it is necessary to increase your dose to ten capsules a day or even more for a couple days; taper off a few capsules daily until you are on the lowest dose necessary to control your symptoms. If you must use higher doses, check your blood pressure and watch your weight. Ideally, have a knowledgeable and understanding physician follow your course.

Adrenal fatigue is a common end result of chronic stress such as chronic illness. In this situation, you are always tired and your blood pressure may run low. A couple daily capsules of licorice

—

may help tremendously by feeding the worn out adrenals especially when taken along with the glandular mullein.

14. Nettle leaf (*Urtica dioica*). If you plan on harvesting your own, be sure to wear gloves as the plant contains stinging hairs that have the highly irritant formic acid. After the plant is either dried thoroughly or cooked, the formic acid is destroyed, removing the irritant component.

    This plant is particularly nutritive as well as anti-inflammatory and anti-histaminic. The entire plant can be used in tea form or tincture and capsule form, and especially in steamed form cooked similarly to spinach. The plant is a blood purifier, stimulating kidney action. Older leaves though may be too strong for the kidneys, so it is best to collect the younger leaves for medicine and food. This plant is extremely safe and can be taken freely.

15. Chamomile, leaves and flowers (*Anthemis nobilis*). This plant is a very useful antispasmodic to the gastrointestinal tract and all muscle groups and is relaxing to the mind as well, making the plant help in anxiety situations. The plant can be especially useful to children. The herb has delicate valuable oils as many do, and thus the tea should be simmered covered to avoid the escape of these volatile oils.

    A note of caution though, although this plant is considered very safe, it is in the ragweed family. Those who are allergic to ragweed may also be allergic to chamomile. Another plant in this family is yarrow. All these can cause reactions, probably about 20 percent or more of those allergic to ragweed will also be allergic to the others. Symptoms may be indigestion or abdominal swelling. The chance for this allergy increases with frequent exposure. Nettle, catnip, and red raspberry would make a suitable, tasty substitute tea.

—

16. Marshmallow root (*Althaea officinalis*). This plant is highly mucilaginous and extremely healing to any inflamed tissues. The powder can be used to pack ulcers and taken internally for ulcerations in the bowel. The root alleviates local irritation, coating the damaged tissue with a protective layer. The plant is full of minerals as evidenced by the deep root system it establishes. Historically, the plant was used for gangrene.

    You can either take the herb as a tea, encapsulated, powdered in a shake or added to the enema. The root is also widely available in tincture form. I recommend the glycerin tincture form as glycerin is nutritive in itself and very well tolerated. It is easy to find this herb in combination with the astragalus available for children. This is especially helpful in the management of children with irritated bowel, as the taste is pleasant and a dropper-full can be easily placed in the juice or herbal tea you feed your child, or yourself for that matter.

17. White oak, inner bark (*Quercus alba*). The powdered bark is highly astringent and anti-inflammatory, helping to stop bleeding as well as restore tissue strength. Oak is not irritating and is safe for use on all tissues. The bark can be quite helpful in assuaging diarrhea, mildly astringing.

    One great unique use of white oak bark is in the treatment of gingivitis. The powder is very restorative to the gums, potentially saving teeth in affected persons. Open the capsule and apply the powder topically at bedtime for weeks, depending on your situation. The powder is perfectly safe. You only need small amounts, one capsule should be sufficient for the entire mouth. It helps pain as well as strengthening gum tissues.

18. Slippery elm, inner bark (*Ulmus rubra*). The inner bark is extremely soothing and nourishing to any damaged tissues. Slippery elm is somewhat similar in activity to marshmallow root but somewhat

—

less irritating, not cleansing, and more nourishing. The powder can be made into gruel by placing the powder in a bowl, adding small amounts of warm water at a time and gentle mixing until thickened then sweetened with honey. Better tolerated than any other food I have heard of, this gruel is quite healing to any tissues it contacts. For those who cannot tolerate any other foods, slippery elm can literally be a lifesaver.

The powder is very easily assimilated into tissue, and can be used on open wounds after careful cleansing as an organic protective layer that will encourage thorough healing. The powder can also be made into a paste to apply to wounds. Also, small amounts of the powder are extremely nourishing in enema fluid. After the tea is prepared, put in a small amount, a teaspoon or so, and blend thoroughly. You do not want the enema tea too thick to pass through the tubing.

A word of caution though, this tree is endangered. The tree should be planted and tended to for the irreplaceable medicinal value alone, much less for the salvation of this species. Use the powder responsibly and try to locate a young tree you can plant.

19. Cascara sagrada root (*Rhamnus purshiana*). This effective laxative can be irritating. The colon motility is enhanced. This plant must be of good quality from a reputable source; the root must be aged at least a year for tolerability—this is routine. The plant has many nutritive substances but should be used in combination with other healing and tonic plants for best effect.

Cascara may be damaging for patients with active inflammation of the intestines and is not recommended for children under the age twelve unless under competent supervision. Small doses used infrequently though can be helpful and safe for children. This plant is extremely useful as a mild laxative in elderly

—

or adult patients with constipation to soften stools and improve bowel health.

20. Cayenne (*Capsicum frutescens*). Cayenne is especially helpful in stabilizing circulation. Also, the fruit, powdered and put in massage oils, can be useful for nerve pain applied on the skin. This plant has been used medicinally for at least nine thousand years. Patients who have poor circulation or neuropathy should benefit from a small daily dose of cayenne, one-two capsules of "cool cayenne" in the morning with a full glass of water can be quite healing over a period of time.

    The activity of cayenne is expressed in heat units or "btu." The higher the btu rating, the hotter the cayenne. Thus cool cayenne has 40,000 btus while "hot" cayenne has 80,000 btus.

    This plant has many valuable nutritional components, including vitamins.

21. Comfrey (*Symphytum officinale*). Although now on the "black list" for internal use, comfrey has such powerful healing properties it must be mentioned. The danger lies in the components called pyrrolizidine alkaloids that can be harmful to an irritated liver. The roots and older leaves contain most of this constituent, the young leaves are the safest for internal use, such as adding comfrey to a "green drink."

    The plant contains allantoin, also in aloe vera, as well as other components that act to speed healing. Allantoin is well established as a cell proliferant. Other constituents certainly play an important role in the dramatic healing effects of comfrey in massage oils or even in green drinks from garden plants.

    The leaves, although slightly irritating when fresh (hairy), can also be boiled and then applied as a poultice for healing wounds, but for those managing bowel disorders, young comfrey leaves in the drinks mentioned above are quite useful.

22. Dandelion (*Taraxacum officinale*). Dandelion is such a valuable "weed," totally misunderstood but important in current lifestyles. Dandelion contains many safe medicinal constituents, especially the inulin, the safe sugar, and the bitter principles deserve mention. The bitters stimulate the liver function, and the many vitamins including a high amount of minerals such as potassium make this plant invaluable in a mixed salad. Inulin is a sugar that is safe and stabilizing for diabetic patients; burdock also contains this component.

The plant is extremely safe, cleansing and nourishing to both the liver and the kidneys. The plant has been traditionally used in the treatment of liver disease, kidney disease, and diabetes. This herb has diuretic properties that are quite powerful. For those who know that diuretics usually causes a loss of potassium, this plant works as effectively as some pharmaceuticals and contains plenty of potassium in an organic form that protects the patient from potassium loss.

As with many herbs, all the constituents work together as a whole; however, this is lost when we try to extract out one component to the exclusion of the others. The constituents are well known to balance each other, a quality no pharmaceutical can match. Appreciate pharmaceuticals have their place, and they and herbals are not the same. Better health is the goal of both.

Be aware, avoid chemical fertilizers and pesticides where you collect your salad greens.

23. Echinacea (*Echinacea augustifolia*). This plant is well known for the immune stimulation by increasing the number and function of white blood cells. This potentially is not an herb for use in inflammatory conditions because of this effect. I have noted a worsening of my symptoms with the use of the herb. No adverse events have been reported regarding autoimmune events, but there

—

have been reports of echinacea causing rashes. This may be more due to the powerful cleansing effect of echinacea rather than the immune stimulation. Historically, echinacea was (and still is) a blood cleanser, and certainly toxins are released from remote areas such as fat and other tissue deposits certainly could come out the skin as a rash.

The herb is a powerful and effective blood purifier, and this is why I would recommend this plant most readily, even for those with autoimmunity. Insect and snake poisonings would greatly be relieved with generous use of echinacea, along with milk thistle.

This herb is available in many forms, capsules, teas, tinctures both glycerin and alcohol. The glycerin tincture is obviously more tolerated by children and those with intestinal disorders. For effectiveness in immune stimulation, you must use the plant several times a day, for poisonings using a large amount (a two ounce bottle of glycerin tincture) a couple times should help your situation tremendously.

24. Fig leaves and fruit (*Ficus carica*). Not only are the fruits wonderful and valuable medicinally, but the leaves are healing as well. This plant has anti-inflammatory, anticarcinogenic, and analgesic (pain relieving) properties that in addition have a wide variety of uses that include protecting the liver, strengthening the immune system, and pulling out metals from the body. The plant also has constituents helpful for eye health (especially lutein.) The wide variety of uses of this tree makes it a must for any person's garden, and the fruit should be a regular part of the healthful diet. The fruit is especially healing to the digestive system.

The leaves can be bruised and used as a poultice for wounds or made into a tea. The leaves do contain compounds called psoralens which, although are anti-cancer, are well known to increase the skin's sensitivity to the sun when used in tea form, or in otherwise

—

large amounts, allowing for severe sunburn if appropriate precautions are not heeded while you are discovering the value of this plant.

25. Flaxseed (*Linum usitatissimum*) Flaxseed is one of the oldest cultivated plants used for clothes, food, and medicine. Pliny the Elder used flaxseed very commonly in his remedies. The oil and ground seed is extremely helpful in replacing essential fatty acids. This plant has gentle laxative properties and is very soothing to the intestinal lining. The oil is strongly anti-inflammatory.

You can buy whole flaxseeds, set them in pure cold water overnight refrigerated, and then crush them and use them in gruel or added to a shake. Be sure to take the crushed seeds with plenty of pure water.

The oil should be refrigerated as well as it contains the same delicate essential fatty acids. This oil, as with other essential fatty acids, is very important for the development and health of the nervous system, as well as skin and all other tissues. Flaxseed has proven anticarcinogenic effects. Also, the plant is useful in treating lupus nephritis, reducing hardened arteries in at-risk patients, and improving circulation. The oil and crushed seed are specific though for any inflammatory conditions, especially inflammatory bowel. You cannot get too much of this valuable oil, and ten or more capsules a day or a tablespoon or two daily is not unreasonable when inflammatory symptoms are severe or when skin is in severe condition (such as severe eczema.)

26. Garlic (*Allium sativum*). Although better known for the circulatory benefits, garlic's benefits consume the entire body. The food is useful in infection with its antibacterial, antifungal, and antiviral activities.

The sulfur in garlic is strongly antioxidant and anti-inflammatory, meaning it is protective to cells. The sulfur-containing components help scavenge free radicals, the cause of aging and cellular damage. There is also much nutritional value in garlic.

27. Ginkgo biloba (*Ginkgo biloba*). This amazing tree is one of the oldest living plants today; the tree can live over a thousand years. The leaves must be concentrated for medicinal value, the herb should be standardized to 24 percent of the flavonol glycosides. This means fifty pounds of leaves make one pound of concentrated herb.

   The standardized herb is protective to the nervous system, stimulating cellular health and renewal as well as improving circulation. The herb also benefits circulation in other parts of the body and should be used whenever circulatory issues are of concern, along with cayenne. Ginkgo can treat inner ear problems, altitude sickness, and motion sickness as well.

   There are proven studies showing the improvement in mental function in patients with dementia, although the studies are mixed. Ginkgo is very important for getting out of the brain fog that occurs with serious chronic illness. Ginkgo also shows promise with attention deficit disorder both in children and adults. Ginkgo thins blood by decreasing platelet clotting, so do not use if blood pressure is elevated. Increased doses increase this risk. The daily dosage is best divided in two or three doses for a total of 120-240 mg of the standard herb. You can take a single dose in the morning. There have been rare reports of allergic reactions to ginkgo. This is an impressive herb for supporting and protecting mental function and circulation. Quality makes a difference. Start low and increase as needed.

28. Gotu kola (*Centella asiatica*). Another great herb, this plant is very useful for encouraging effective wound healing by stimulating collagen synthesis. The herb also is calming and healing to the nervous system and works well with ginkgo.

29. Ginger (*Zingiber officinale*) Ginger contains many volatile oils, so must be protected with a lid when preparing the root in tea. Ginger is warming, stimulating to the circulation, and improves digestion. The herb is considered "diffusive" going to the heart and then spreading throughout the body, especially the abdominal and pelvic regions.

The tea, prepared by removing the bark from the fresh root and allowed to simmer in other herbal tea blends such as red raspberry leaves, is very useful for nausea and can be helpful to babies, as well as others, with colic, indigestion, and diarrhea. The root is well known to encourage digestion, is antispasmodic, and minimizes griping pains from diarrhea.

Candied ginger is often commercially available and delicious, still having the benefit of soothing indigestion. Ginger can also be chewed fresh after the bark has been peeled.

Although extremely useful for many people suffering nausea and indigestion, it may not be well tolerated by those who have trouble with heat conditions, such as those with inflammatory bowel or peptic ulcers. If it does not make you feel better, do not use it. In these situations, stay with red raspberry leaf tea for nausea and indigestion.

30. Hyssop leaves (*Hyssopus officinalis*). This mild herb benefits the lungs, circulation, kidneys, as well as the intestines. The herb is specific for "damp mucus" conditions, such as conditions associated with indigestion, appetite loss, abdominal distension and pain, and chills. The herb also is antiparasitic. Deficiency symptoms with long-term fatigue and depression are replenished and warmed, as hyssop is a yang tonic, deeply warming and strengthening. Hyssop has an uplifting effect on the spirit because of its nervous restorative properties.

Hyssop has powerful antiseptic properties and is quite helpful in enema form to stimulate liver function and detoxification. The herb is also quite useful as a wash for wounds as tea; it is quite gentle.

The essential oil of hyssop contains a potentially toxic ketone called pino-camphene and therefore should only be used on a limited basis. If the oil is used, take only one-two drops in a small glass of water for a short term, as over time there is risk for seizures. The herb is also contraindicated during pregnancy because it stimulates the uterus.

31. Gravel root (*Eupatorium purpureum*). Also known as queen of the meadow, gravel root is very useful in dissolving calcifications throughout the body. Stones in various places, as well as adhesions within the abdomen, may all be softened and potentially relieved with the regular use of gravel root.

    Gravel root has cooling and astringing qualities and has been historically used in kidney disorders, neuralgias, and rheumatism. The herb is extremely soothing and may help relax nerves in some individuals. Also, the herb supports a healthy immune system.

    The herb is best medicinally as an alcoholic tincture; the medicinal compounds are more readily made available. The alcohol tincture can be used safely in bowel complaints by allowing the alcohol to be evaporated off by placing the tincture in hot tea.

32. Lobelia (*Lobelia inflata*). This is a unique herb, valuable in almost if not all formulas. Dr. Christopher called this plant the "thinking herb." In low doses, lobelia leaves calm nausea; in large doses, lobelia is an emetic, meaning it causes vomiting.

    Lobelia is what got Samuel Thompson in trouble in the 1800s because of a prank he played. He gave a large amount of lobelia to an unsuspecting victim and caused a lot of vomiting. Thompson was accused of trying to kill the person. You could not take in enough lobelia by mouth to cause death; it would also be pounds injected to kill a person. Lobelia is safe in usual doses.

33. Lemon balm (*Melissa officinalis*). This plant is especially soothing, tastes good in tea form as well as being available in glycerin tinctures suitable especially for children. The plant is highly aromatic, so again steep the tea in a lidded pan. The herb helps with nervousness, spasms, and insomnia. It also contains anti-inflammatory, antibiotic, and antiviral properties, making its value important in any home medicine chest. The plant has a history of use for herpes infections. The plant is in the mint family, helping to explain the value in alleviating nausea.

There is a study alleging that the plant over a period of time impairs thyroid function, so caution must be taken in the use of the plant over extended periods of time. The studies were outside of the body and are purely speculative. Because thyroid disease is so prevalent now, I worry more about purifying your water supply than taking too much Melissa.

This plant grows quite easily and returns yearly to add much fragrance to the garden.

34. Milk thistle (*Silybum marianum*). This desperately needed plant is best concentrated to a standardized level of 70-80 percent silymarin, thought to be the most active constituent. The plants seeds contain these medicinal properties, valuable in healing liver complaints of all kinds. The spleen, kidneys, and gastrointestinal tract also benefit from milk thistle; this is not just a liver remedy, although the most important use is here.

Milk thistle improves liver function primarily in two ways, by preventing toxins from entering liver cells and by stimulating liver cell regeneration (renewal.) The herb is indicated for liver disease of all types, with significant benefit in liver regeneration and function over time. The German Commission E, a standard of herbal literature, finds no known interactions with the use of milk thistle. There are also no known contraindications, factors that make it harmful to use the plant. Improvement in liver function is well documented.

The concentrated extract is the preferred form because silymarin is poorly water soluble, making it difficult to use medicinally in tea. The dose of concentrated extract is fifteen-twenty-five drops four-five times a day or 100-200 mg silymarin equivalent capsules twice daily. This plant must be taken for several months for obvious benefit. There is clinical experience to suggest the seeds help arthritis as well, supporting the role in detoxification as a beneficial factor in arthritis.

35. Parsley (*Petroselinum sativum*). This plant contains valuable diuretic properties. It is also rich in vitamins and minerals such as iron, potassium, and calcium, as well as vitamin C and A. Parsley is useful for supporting kidney function and aiding in the release of stones from the kidney as well as gallbladder.

The plant is nutritive and can easily be added to carrot juice or green drinks. Eating a sprig or two of parsley also is beneficial. The plant is thought to be helpful in preventing cancer with the high organic potassium content as well as other valuable constituents.

You should not use the plant if you are suffering from a kidney infection; this could irritate the already stressed organs.

36. Shepherd's purse (*Capsella bursa-pastoris*). This plant is primarily useful in the first aid kit for any bleeding problems. The herb is available in alcohol tincture form. One-two dropper-full quite effectively stops a nosebleed of any degree. Gastrointestinal bleeding certainly will stop with the use of this medicine as well. The benefit is obvious and dramatic. Caution might be used in patients at risk for stroke, but in general, those who are bleeding are not having stroke at the same time. Use the medicine only

—

when needed. Save it for these times. There is no other plant like this one.

37. Thyme (*Thymus vulgaris*). This plant has powerful antiseptic as well as relaxant properties. Thyme benefits not only nervous conditions but also people with respiratory complaints with its decongestant, expectorant, and relaxant properties. This plant is a good remedy for those with a weak stomach due to indigestion and cramps, and stimulates liver function as well.

In addition to being antiseptic, which is important for infectious processes, the plant also is a diuretic, which helps relieve fluid retention. The plant in tea form is warm and drying, restoring, astringing, and stimulating to the body as a whole.

The essential oil is highly concentrated and should be diluted in fresh oil such as safflower or sweet almond oil for massage.

38. Violet *(Viola odorata)*. This plant is available in many forms and tastes well in tea blends. Violet flowers and leaves are calming and pain relieving with anti-inflammatory properties. The plant also is a valuable blood purifier.

39. Black walnut (*Juglans nigra*). Black walnut husks are extremely valuable in combination treatments for parasites. Black walnut is also antifungal, helping to resolve yeast and other fungal infections.

Black walnut contains organic iodine. Some people develop allergy to this.

40. Wormwood (*Artemisia absinthium*). This plant is also an important antiparasitic medicine. Use in low doses, one cup of tea day for an adult, less in children. This herb is best tolerated in capsule or tincture form taken according to label instructions.

Wormwood historically was abused in liquor as an intoxicant (absinthe). The use of this liquor was banned after many suffered irreversible brain damage from the abuse of the beverage. Use the herb with care, and do not abuse it and cause it to be removed from our antiparasitic armamentarium.

41. White pond lily (*Nymphaea odorata*). This plant is helpful in pain management. It is healing to inflamed tissues as well as lung troubles. The plant is soothing to the gastrointestinal tract as well as the kidney passageways. The plant is excellent for children with bowel complaints. White pond lily also makes a great poultice for wounds, abscesses, and skin lesions.

42. Yarrow (*Achillea milliafolium*). This is a very bitter herb whose flowering tops have wonderful detoxifying and diaphoretic (cause sweating) properties. This allows the release of toxins out the pores effectively. Be sure to drink plenty of fluids while encouraging the sweating process. Hot bathes are sufficient to encourage sweating in addition to the use of yarrow.

    The plant is also significantly anti-inflammatory. The plant is usually drunk in tea form, but because it is so bitter, it is better tolerated either in capsule form or in tea for enema use.

    Use this herb in small amounts for enema preparation; the herb is astringing (drying out). It is a great liver aid; when used in enema form, it greatly clears nausea as well as allergies. For those with bowel complaints including nausea, yarrow may be used in enema preparations; hyssop is a gentler substitute. A little goes a long way. Powerful herbs may be more sensitizing so use with care.

    Because the herb is so detoxifying, do not use the plant during pregnancy. Also watch for allergy to yarrow as it is sensitizing.

43. Yellow dock (*Rumex crispus*). This plant is also widely available, growing wild throughout much of the United States. The plant is helpful in detoxification and stimulates liver activity quite effectively. Also, the plant is nourishing, containing minerals such as organic iron. The root contains berberine, a known antibiotic that stimulates liver activity. This is considered the active

—

constituent of goldenseal. I do not recommend goldenseal by the way because the plant is seriously endangered and should not be taken orally because it does not absorbed well. Goldenseal is a wonderful wash and drying antiseptic agent for wounds but should be limited to this use.

Because the plant contains a large amount of tannins, which are drying, you should limit the use of the plant to every other week at most.

There are so many useful herbs not mentioned above; this list is by no means all-inclusive. This list only suggests some of the more useful herbs for digestion and related issues.

CHAPTER 18

Adverse Interactions, Allergies, and Sensitivities to Natural Therapies and Reactions with Pharmaceutical Medications

Because of the return of herbal medicine supported with greater scientific knowledge, undesirable actions are recognized more frequently. Although the adverse reactions in people are not nearly as frequent by any stretch of the imagination as pharmaceutical's adverse reactions, we do not have adequately trained healers to monitor appropriately for this possibility. Medically trained physicians usually are not trained to understand the nuances of herbs and generally do not understanding the mechanism of herbs, causing herbs to become a sort of scapegoat for any adverse reaction a patient might experience. Therefore, it is difficult to interpret the literature. Confounding this is the pharmaceutical industries' attempts to control the market and their profits. Herbs cannot be patented, so either you come up with some magic bullet as an answer to disease from constituents extracted from plants or you chemically synthesize a drug that you can patent. Medicines in the form of whole herbs are generally not profitable, especially those that can be grown in any backyard garden. These are in fact the medicines with the most potential, as long as people are educated to the use of herbs, for medicines grown easily in our environment must be the most economical. There is a serious problem with accepting garden plants as having medicinal value. Who will pay the expense for the clinical trials necessary to prove their usefulness? Who will study the uses these plants have to determine their potential risks? Understanding these limitations, it becomes increasingly clear we must study the knowledge already gained by our healing forefathers; for example, Hippocrates himself used many of the herbs we use today. What were his experiences and results? What about great healers such as Nicholas Culpepper and Jethro Kloss? What about the obvious successes of people such as John Christopher? Do not assume all folklore and historical medicine as having no basis in science, for they are showing over and over in current clinical trials the accuracy of many of the historical of herbs. These herbs were quite useful then and even possibly more so now. We have even more reasons to require cleansing and detoxification programs as our world becomes increasingly toxic. Unfortunately, politics and money have thwarted much of the advances in herbal medicine. Now, because of the money going into herbal products, the industry is under jeopardy of making false promises and causing pain and suffering as people compete and scurry to get the next magic bullet. Integrity is so important in any healing industry, and I hope natural healers can be happy making an honest living rather than falling into greed like has happened so many times in our past.

It is important to know to both the good and bad of herbs. We must stay open minded. As I stated before, we cannot possibly know all the effects because each person is unique and our environment is much different than that of the past. We have different genetic weaknesses, different nutritional deficiencies, and a much different environment. Therefore, it is important for you to respect personal traits that may cause you to respond in a particular way. You also must learn to trust your instinct, your inner voice. Do not be so fixed in your opinions that you do not grow. Learning is continuous; don't cling to understandings from your past but allow them to evolve.

One of the most important suggestions I can make regarding herbs and foods is to smell them or take a small taste. Listen to your intuition and your senses. Obviously some herbs like valerian stink, so you should not go just on that basis. This may be a way valerian protects children from being attracted to the relaxing plant. Valerian might attract those requiring its medicine although the smell will still stink. What I have found is the smell isn't quite so repulsive to those needing valerian. If it is in a capsule, break it open. If you are not drawn to an herb, there is a chance it is not good for you. I know this kind of sounds mystical, but bear with me. Learn to trust your inner wisdom most of all. If you can find someone knowledgeable to help you heal, trust your instinct here as well. If you do not trust your physician, chances are you will not have a healing encounter.

Plants are well known to cause problems with bleeding. In general, stop all herbs for at least a week or two at best prior to any surgery. Here is a list of some of the most common offenders.

Bleeding

Herbs known or suspected for increasing bleeding tendencies:

1. Alfalfa (blood thinner, purifier)
2. Boswellia (anti-inflammatory)
3. Capsaicin (circulatory stimulant)
4. Clovers, yellow, red, or white (blood thinner)
5. Don Quai
6. Dan Shen

7. Garlic (inhibits platelets)
8. Ginkgo biloba (circulatory antioxidant)
9. Green tea (inhibits platelets)
10. Licorice root (anti-inflammatory)
11. Meadowsweet (salicylate anti-inflammatory)
12. St. John's wort (purifier)
13. Turmeric (anti-inflammatory COX-2)
14. White willow bark (salicylate)

If you use these herbs on a regular basis and find you greatly benefit from them, do not be afraid of them. If you have an injury, just hold a little extra pressure, their increased risk of bleeding is very small. The problem arises when you combine these herbs with stronger pharmaceutical medications that also promote bleeding. Obviously this can be a problem. If your teeth bleed easily or you cannot get small cuts to stop within a reasonable time with ample pressure, you may be having a problem. Stop or at least slow the herbs down. Go with much lower dosages; see if you get the medicinal value without the side effect from a lower dose. If the bleeding is prolonged, you should have it further evaluated by a physician. But try shepherd's purse which might reverse the bleeding tendency. Shepherd's purse can stop bleeding but use with caution as shepherds purse may increase blood clots. A half dropper in a small glass of water is usually sufficient to stop a bleed. Although I have found cayenne on bleeding tendency lists, I am not convinced of the accuracy of chili peppers to increase the risk of bleeding. Historically and by experience, I have found capsaicin stops or controls bleeding and would recommend it for such.

There are potential interactions with pharmaceutical medications. Many herbal contraindications are based solely on theoretical concerns. Keep herbs in moderate usage, more is not necessarily better.

Pharmaceutical interactions:

Many herbs are suspected or known to interact with pharmaceutical drugs. A common example of this interaction is herbs with monoamine-oxidase inhibitor (MAOI) pharmaceutical drugs. Herbs have very weak MAO inhibitor activity in themselves, but when combined with certain medications, this can be a very serious problem. Monoamine-oxidase is an enzyme system located throughout our body but especially in our brain. This enzyme system is responsible for the breakdown of neurochemicals such as serotonin. Therefore, MAO inhibitors allow for a rise in serotonin levels in the brain. Antidepressants in the MAO inhibitor class are extremely vulnerable to interactions with herbs as well as many other pharmaceuticals. In general, we do not prescribe these type medications anymore because of this risk. When combined with interactive medications, either herbal or pharmaceutical, serious problems such as high blood pressure can result. Basically, herbs that affect liver enzymes can potentiate MAO inhibitors. These include gingko (speculative), St. John's wort, and California poppy. Stimulating herbs containing caffeine such as cocoa, coffee, cola, guarana, and ma huang (ephedra) can all be harmful combined with MAO inhibitor antidepressants. I don't recommend their use because of their draining effect on the physical body in general, especially to the adrenals. Remember, just because something is organic or plant based does not mean it is healthful. It is much better to build up the body so adaptations are easily made rather than over-stimulate an already exhausted body. Build up a reserve, get the rest and nutrition you need and be patient. Only use caffeinated herbs on a limited basis, especially if you suffer from chronic disease. Also, certain herbs, specifically ginseng, can potentiate MAO inhibitors, causing manic like symptoms in susceptible individuals. Be extra cautious if any pharmaceutical medication you take contains

MAO inhibitors. Pharmaceuticals have much more pronounced activity than herbs, so do not worry if you are not on these medications.

Another potential herb-drug interaction occurs when you take supportive nourishing herbs while you are treating symptoms of the disease process. As the tissues heal, you may become more responsive to the pharmaceutical medications requiring lower dosages. An example, although not necessarily borne out in literature, might be hawthorn berry healing heart tissue, causing increased responsiveness to heart medications. I advise continuing the healing herb while monitoring your response carefully. For example, if your blood pressure improves, lower your blood pressure medication. This obviously needs the support of your family doctor. Remember, you are not taking hawthorn to substitute a drug to control symptoms, you are aiming at helping the underlying cause. This will take time. It took you a long time to get in the situation you are in, it will take some time getting you out. Find a physician knowledgeable and supportive. Garlic might also improve heart health, cholesterol, etc., thus necessitating lower pharmaceutical doses. This is good.

Allergic Reactions to Herbs

This is becoming a more common problem, as our immune systems become increasingly "dysfunctional" and our bowel is increasingly "leaky." I have not found this to be a recognized problem in the distant past, leading me to assume environmental changes to play a major role in the development of allergies and intolerances. Likely the most commonly recognized sensitizing herb is chamomile. This plant is of the composite or aster family, so if you have problems with this plant, it is wise to use caution with other plants in this family, namely yarrow and wormwood. Ragweed is also a member of this family. In these cases, smell the herb first and consider your reaction and intuition. Often we develop sensitivities over a period of time, so just because you have taken the herb without a problem in the past does not excuse you from a current problem. Symptoms can include swelling, itching, and general intestinal distress to breathing problems and obstructive symptoms. Do not ignore these symptoms that may be subtle. If you get them, seek the advice of a physician; if mild, take some licorice root and frequent small amounts of liquids, holding off on meals until symptoms are resolving. This may be one case where herbs such as ma huang have a place in therapy, but it is much more prudent to seek outside help in the case of moderate to severe allergy.

Psyllium husks are also known to be sensitizing, possibly by virtue of its irritant qualities. Flaxseed gruel may be a much better alternative. Tannins in various herbs can be sensitizing as well because of their very astringent action. Keep this in mind as you choose your therapy. Also, herbs that are more commonly recommended without addressing the entire situation of leaky bowel and inflammation potentially could be more sensitizing as you use these herbs on inflamed tissues. For example, I became sensitive to goldenseal from chronic exposure in an herbal blend I was taking to manage bowel symptoms. Always consider healing the inflammation in gentle ways, restoring the integrity of the bowel. Also, work on getting your liver functioning efficiently, as a healthy liver also is necessary to control and prevent sensitization. A healthy liver more adequately removes sensitizing proteins from your bloodstream, minimizing exposure. Work on hyper-immunity by minimizing exposures of known allergens, toxins, and other waste products. Parasites and yeasts also may play a significant role in hypersensitivity that should be addressed. With bowel disease, you are at higher risk for developing food and herb sensitivities. If allergy occurs, consider licorice root or astragalus and marshmallow root to calm the immune system. See a physician if breathing problems or severe reactions occur. This may also be a situation calling for ma huang, a rare situation. Ma huang and similar stimulating herbs open up the lungs but have a potential for racing the heart. Use judiciously. Always use stimulating herbs with much caution.

Other Herbal Toxicities

Another potential problem with herbs may occur if you take herbs that place too much demand on one or more organ systems. For example, as previously mentioned, caffeine in a variety of plants over-stimulates the adrenal as well as the heart, potentially causing further aggravation of disease processes. The vasoconstriction associated with stimulants such as caffeine also can cause problems with circulation causing ischemia that can be very harmful. Without adequate blood supply, tissues cannot fulfill their function, regenerate effectively, and even die off. Obviously this can be a problem that can be acutely serious or chronically insidious depending on the dosage and the patient's sensitivity. Some herbs have received a lot of bad publicity because of the over-stimulation to organs; for example, comfrey can place excessive demands on the liver. You must understand comfrey, and if you have liver disease, you should only use comfrey topically where most of the herb bypasses action by the liver. The root of comfrey has more of the potential toxic substances and especially should be avoided by those suspected as having liver disease in any form. But comfrey is still a wonderful plant, very useful in augmenting healing tissues. Another example is juniper berries, very useful for kidney disease. Large doses of juniper berries, and uva ursi as well, have been implicated for being responsible for kidney inflammation. Be sure you do not use these herbs in extreme doses, and be sure the patient gets plenty of beneficial fluids as well. Basically, be aware of the possibility of placing excessive demands on ailing organs and thus potentially worsening their function. Always, start low and go slow.

When you are in the process of healing, always remember to nourish effectively. Do not expect an ailing gastrointestinal system to extract nutrients from complex foods such as meat and pizza, but simplify your food choices to carrot juice or celery juice to provide nourishment as well as support cleansing processes.

Some herbs may cause a "healing crisis" in another way. Here I am referring to antiparasitics, antifungals, and antibiotics that may cause an elevated load of dead products that your body must clear. This is especially true with antiparasitics, which are rarely used in our culture thus resulting in heavy parasite burdens. You may feel very ill if you too rapidly kill off these menaces, and this potentially could be very dangerous if you are already weak and deficient. As previously stated, start low and go slow. Drink plenty of fluids and especially keep your bowels moving when taking antiparasitics in particular. You want to pass the parasites rather than let them putrefy, leading to autointoxication. Realize that you may not feel well on the antiparasitics early on, but you will get increasingly stronger and feel increasingly better as you persist in this case. The healing crisis should become less frequent and less severe as you continue your program for health. If this is not the case, something is getting missed so seek out appropriate qualified help whenever you can.

I wish you the best in finding your health and your purpose in life. I hope you will continue to seek out truth regarding health and the care of our physical bodies. I pray you will be inspired by my experiences and expertise and be able to incorporate these lifestyle practices with understanding and ease. Remember, healing is somewhat a slow process, but it is possible. This is a hard process most times, but the results of better vitality and a clearer spirit are worth the sacrifices. Don't stay shackled to your poor health. Seek and apply knowledge and wisdom to your abilities. I wish you health.

Appendix A

Disclosure for Complimentary Medicine Approaches

There are various methods of healing throughout the world. I have studied historical herbal and complimentary approaches and philosophies such as those found in Chinese medicine. Keep in mind this is not "evidenced-based medicine," as the studies require significant costs, and many of my suggestions you may be able to grow in your own backyard. Please understand, I have preference for native plants and foods. I do not comparatively know Chinese herbs, I generally recommend our own native plants in most instances, plants that are natural to our environments. However, Chinese medicine philosophy keeps me interested. Combining herbal and nutritional practices with standard medical approaches offers benefits to health.

I do consider myself an authority on natural healing. As such, at times I may recommend non-Western but still traditional approaches to promote healing. My most basic philosophy is to provide the body what it needs to heal, the building blocks. In most cases, this is a large component to healing. Nutrients, pure water, herbal remedies, all can be much source of our "fountain of youth." I am not here to improve your lifespan, as I do not believe I have that power, but I can help you with gaining a better quality life with healthful living as well as medical care. Hippocrates used some of the very same plants I suggest. And his phrase, "Do no harm," is timeless.

As a result of much confusion, complimentary medicine generally is not supported by medical insurance. Office visits for complimentary healing at this time are not reimbursed by medical insurance companies in most states.

Warnings regarding complimentary approaches:

1. Do not believe everything you read, hear, or see. There are still a lot of "snake oils" and get-rich-quick schemes.
2. Buy quality, pay attention to brands. There is a large variation in quality of herbal and nutraceutical nutrients. There has been concern regarding purity of products as well.

Appendix B

Herbal teas

Many herbs can be useful for alleviating suffering and discomfort. I have come to rely on them on a regular basis to keep my own family healthy. When my children are ill, herbs are the first medication I reach for because of their extreme safety and benefit when used skillfully. With any bowel condition, herbs are the standard in management, for they encourage healing by calming inflammation, nourishing, stimulating and protecting cells, and strengthening tissues. Herbs are uniquely qualified for preventing, treating, and healing our bodies.

Useful teas for overall strengthening, toning, and healing include various combinations with a base of red raspberry leaf tea. I find this tea very nourishing as well as flavorful and refreshing. Red raspberry is very nutritious. The constituents are mildly astringent and cleansing as well as support the elasticity of collagen. Iron, neutral vitamin C in the leaf is very easy to digest and assimilate.

Generally, I combine three or four teabags of red raspberry leaf with a couple other nutritional tea bags to a 4—or 6-quart pan of boiling pure water. Bring purified water to a boil, add the teabags of choice, turn off and cover to simmer. Some considerations to use might include combinations of the following, but options are endless.

1) Catnip leaf—nervine, antispasmodic, relaxant
2) Chamomile—nervine, antispasmodic, relaxant, cousin of ragweed so use small amounts
3) Elderberry, Bilberry—antiviral and antioxidant, especially for eyes
4) Hawthorn berry—very useful in anxiety, heart conditions of all kinds, and calming
5) Echinacea—blends well with others, blood cleansing—use periodically for immune stimulation, caution with autoimmune illnesses.
6) Nettle leaf (dried)—very nutritional, tastes well, caution with fresh plant, stinging nettle
7) Peppermint leaf—tastes well, relaxing to the bowels, but can be somewhat stimulating and might not be used near bedtime
8) Hyssop, purifying, "cleanse me with hyssop, I will be white as snow." This is biblical.

When you prepare these teas, you also can use purified or distilled water. Distilled water has the added advantage of being devoid of any minerals, making this water "hungry." I do have concern for distilled bottled water though, as the plastics have their own chemical components that are not beneficial. You can purchase a distiller for the best purification of water. This hungry water is prepared by bringing purified water to steam and then collecting that steam and reconstituting it into water. Distilled water picks up more nutrients from the teas because it is empty aside from its own molecules, making herbal teas prepared with this water more nutritive, and up to 30 percent more effective according to reliable experts on the field of natural healing. Indeed, I have noticed increased benefit of using distilled water. Purified water does well though, and triple water filters can provide water free from chlorine, minerals, and other contaminants in our usually public water supply. This water has its own minerals and does not pick up the nutrients from the teas quite so readily, but still is sufficient in making a good healthful tea.

Another consideration is many of these healthful teas contain extremely volatile essential oils as part of their active constituents. Therefore, these teas should be covered and not brought to a boil for long, in an effort to preserve these valuable oils in the tea. After you prepare these teas adequately, you will notice the oil droplets collecting on the surface of the prepared tea; this lets you know the teas were prepared correctly with the retention of these valuable oils. Indeed, you will not notice nearly as much benefit if you prepare these teas uncovered or boiled too aggressively. Chamomile, catnip, and other nervine quality teas are particularly delicate and should be prepared in a somewhat gentle way, especially covered while brewing and storing the hot tea. Much medicinal value can be lost as vapor to the air. If you doubt what I am saying, try comparing uncovered and covered chamomile tea of the same initial quality. Catnip tea is not as tasty, so combining this with raspberry tea allows improved taste. Sometimes you might doubt the benefits of the particular herb or supplement, when the herb was improperly prepared or stored, or collected for that matter. It is important to get the highest quality herbs you can, and herbs of questionable quality are generally not worth taking at all.

Appendix C

Calcium

Calcium is a very important mineral for our bone health as well as other functions, such as the muscular system. It is important to supply our body with natural wholesome ideally plant-chelated calcium. The best form of calcium is incorporated into plants. Blackstrap molasses is loaded with calcium, as well as other valuable minerals in a plant bonded form. Unfortunately, blackstrap molasses' taste requires adjustment, and I recommend 1 tablespoon three times a week chased with orange juice or other juice. Blackstrap is loaded in magnesium and potassium as well as others. Renal patients may need less. Blackstrap is the byproduct of sugar cane, all the minerals removed to make white sugar. You can only get this in health food stores. Regular molasses in most grocery stores is only flavored like blackstrap but not the same. Blackstrap molasses supports healing as a super nutrient. I have witnessed people steadily and dramatically heal from all sorts of injuries and illnesses. Effect on osteoporosis is likely the most obvious and reliable benefit, but other problems such as diabetes, neurological, and heart disease also respond favorably with blackstrap. I have been told it tastes like barbecue sauce. I often tell people it tastes like bad cough syrup until the barbecue sauce association was made. Start with a teaspoon with a chaser such as juice a day, three times a week.

Other valuable sources of calcium include dark green vegetables, celery, parsley, and possibly coral. Coral calcium is interesting, it alkalinizes very efficiently with the trace minerals associated with coral. The source is the question though, so routinely, I do not recommend coral unless it is from a quality source. Vegetables washed well can easily be juiced with the many user-friendly juicers commercially available. A good habit to develop is a morning juice, as many healthy people have found.

Calcium binds other molecules and thus causes trouble with absorption of vitamins, pharmaceuticals, and other medicines. In addition, calcium is poorly absorbed. It should be taken with a meal for best absorption, but not with supplements and medicines. Calcium on an empty stomach may be only absorbed at 10 percent for example. Take calcium with food to aid the absorption. Also do bone building activities to stimulate the activity of bone formation and thus increase the demand for calcium.

Calcium carbonate is not my favorite form of calcium. Carbonate is chalk or talc. This form may coat the stomach as in Tums formulas, but there are significant concerns. Why do we have so many calcium deposits in places other than the bone. Why does the calcium stay in the bloodstream, or deposit on joints? In any event, my recommendation is to prioritize calcium and get a decent formula. Calcium phosphate and calcium gluconate are possibilities. Renal patients must be cautions though with the phosphate forms. Especially severe renal disease contributes to poor calcium in itself, and quality is so much more important than quantity.

It is very difficult if not possible to avoid calcium carbonate; it is added to many commercial food products such as almond milk and cereals. I recommend keeping the amount of carbonate ingested to a minimum. There is the possibility that carbonate has a cleansing action to the bowel and therefore is not completely harmful. I recommend taking adequate supplementation with meals. Quality calcium sources are so exponential in how they help support bone and other tissue, and if taken properly, it is unclear the actual recommended daily requirements at exactly 1200 mg a day. It depends on the demands the body is under and on effective uptake and assimilation. Walking down the stairs is just as important as walking up. There are many isotonic exercises that assist in encouraging bone formation. Regular exercise obviously is valuable in bone.

Celery is unique for bone. It contains silica which stimulates the bone. Parsley added in modest amounts to juices or tea also contains many trace minerals in plant-bonded form. Healthy glands play a role in healthy bones. Parsley is very good for the adrenal as well as peas and green beans, which again supports bone. Parsley and celery are great to add to home-prepared vegetable and fruit juices.

Vitamin D is necessary for bone health. This fat soluble vitamin is best absorbed taken with omega supplements or other good fats. You're your omega oils and D3 at the same time. Later take calcium with food. Calcium impairs absorption of D vitamin when taken together. There are basically three forms of vitamin D: D1 from diet converted to D2 by kidneys converted to vitamin D3 by the skin with the help of sunlight. D3 is the most active form by a significant amount. D supports bone remodeling and repair and supports the immune system and the nervous system and therefore all systems. Many people live with low D3 levels. I look for this in most individuals. I have seen the D levels improve much better with, rather than without, taking omega oils at the same time as the D3; better absorption is proven in my office. People do feel better with D3 correction, although they are doing other things as well to get better, so I cannot attribute the improved well being solely as a result of D3. I have seen D3 levels in single digits, six or seven probably the lowest but not totally rare. Many levels are in the teens. The normal level is considered 30-100. D2 levels have been normal or even elevated with these very low D3s, suggesting we are not converting D2 to D3 in the skin properly.

This vitamin is not getting converted by the sun properly. The benefit of tanning for mood may be linked to D3 synthesis. Sun exposure is increasingly dangerous, so sunscreen is important. I am not sure sunscreen is the cause as I do not see any association of sunscreen use with low D3 levels. Tanning indeed likely does assist D conversion but the damage to the skin is not worth that benefit. I suspect there are factors in the air that are causing us trouble in converting D2 to D3. I wonder about factors that could impair conversion such as ozone or pollutants. Correct your D3 orally and then take care of the why. Supplementation certainly improves health. Vitamin D also is necessary for good nervous and immune function.

Appendix D

The Medicine Chest

Various plants can offer much in first aid and emergency care. Some relatively inexpensive herbals and oils can be helpful to support healing. Among my favorite are the following:

1. Slippery elm, *Ulmas rubra* inner bark. This is considered to be a fluffy gel that becomes flesh. It of course should be well preserved and clean, and capsules alone can suffice. You can open a capsule on various open wounds. This should be cleaned gently daily and redressed with an oil-based or antibacterial salve with the powder placed on top. The powder as well can be used internally, as it is readily available in capsules. I keep my herbals cool, refrigerated if I can, to prolong their qualities; and slippery elm benefits and lasts years in a cool refrigerator, or even freezer, as long it has been properly dried and kept dry.

2. Eucalyptus oil. I always recommend patch testing a small area of skin first, as this is always the best approach with any complimentary approach to healing. If there is no reaction, then this is wonderful as a chest rub, so much more valuable than

traditional camphor products. Along with bronchodilation, the oil is considered to be antiviral, antiparasitic, and antibacterial by many well-respected traditional and historical healers, i.e., Hippocrates. Do not take this orally. This oil is just so handy in the medicine cabinet.

3. Cool cayenne. This fruit gives you the potency without the heat. Historically, this was used for circulation issues to balance the circulation. It is thought to help stop bleeding. The topical preparation of cayenne will allow for release of a substance, that when released, produces a sensation of heat while actually depleting pain receptor chemicals and thus reducing pain. The dilation effect then helps to relax muscles.

4. Echinacea. For immediate blood cleansing even more than the immune boost, echinacea is thought to have and does have this effect. This is for when someone is coming down with an infection or has gotten poisoned.

5. Milk thistle. In addition to a treatment to poisoning, it is my first recommendation for liver support of important cleansing functions. Silymarin, considered the most active constituent, should be concentrated, and I believe there are some good resources for quality product. The liver needs all the support it can get. I would even use this in case of chemical exposures as well.

6. Shepherd's purse, *Capsella bursa-pastoris*. For bleeding issues, this in the form of a tincture is amazing. Nosebleeds beware. Used historically for hemorrhage. I would suspect the medicine could be risky for clotting issues, so obviously should be respected for what it is for. I do not think for a bleeding person who is not also clotting somewhere would be fine with a dropper-full of tincture in water a couple times if necessary.

7. Licorice root provides a cortisone base and is quite effective as a prednisonelike plant. This is a major anti-inflammatory herb.

—

The root can raise blood pressure, blood sugar, and cause fluid retention just like prednisone. I doubt is the immune suppressant properties are as pronounced compared to prednisone. In fact, the body's natural cortisol is supported, so possibly licorice root even improves immune function. Can be used in tea as well as in a traditional capsule and tincture forms or raw.

8. Mullen as a capsule or tincture for lung and gland repair. The plant has been used for centuries. I am sure Hippocrates liked mullen.

9. White oak bark for gums, tooth injuries, and for gum support. Can be used with clove or stevia or both. White oak is strengthening to tissues it gives contact to. You may open the capsule and apply directly onto the affected gums and teeth. Leave on for sleep.

10. Olive oil, wheat germ oil, castor oil, all for topical healing. Olive and wheat germ oil are nutritional. Wheat germ oil is full of natural vitamin E. Castor oil is very softening and can be very soothing. Castor oil should never be taken internally though, as it is too strong for the inner lining of the gastrointestinal system.

11. White willow bark would be a blood thinner; this is an aspirin.

12. Red raspberry leaf tea not only as a drink but a wash. This is very gentle, slightly astringing and nourishing.

Appendix E

Echinacea

Echinacea is considered an immune enhancer in current literature. Historically, however, this plant is quite a blood purifier. The plant was used countless years for envenomization, poisonings, etc. Of course, I would add milk thistle to such a harsh poisoning in effort to protect the liver, but please understand the value of echinacea as a blood purifier.

When you cleanse blood, all organs of elimination, i.e., the bowels, kidneys, pores, lungs, and liver must work together as well as possible. The blood needs these organs of elimination to help remove the released toxins. There are various unique properties to the herbal and nutritional cleansers. Watermelon is a great example of a very cleansing food but could be cooling and therefore weakening to certain constitutions. The intensity of the blood purifier should be respected.

There are more gentle blood purifiers, thus safer in certain situations. Red raspberry leaves, those who know me know this tea, is very safe and has valuable blood purification properties. Up the scale would include hyssop and red clover. Red clover I consider a more powerful remedy. Wheatgrass tends to be a gentle cleanser and nourishing to all the organ systems.

My point with echinacea is in its value with vaccines. Echinacea, with all its good reports and studies, is undoubtedly helpful to stimulate the immune system. This plant should not harm the usefulness of the vaccine. But there are no formal studies to confirm, and no problems to reported. Echinacea should be used with the active infection anyway in most cases, so it should help with immune response for vaccines too. On the other hand, the plant is so very valuable as a blood purifier, would it help alleviate the side effects we so fear as parents? In my experience, I use echinacea in glycerin tincture both before and after vaccines. It may just be treating me, but I have not had a single severe reaction from a vaccine since, and I can name off at least a handful prior on my own family. The only possible risk would be if there was allergy to echinacea, so you should probably know this before you go with the vaccine use. This is not standard of care, this is a naturopathic perspective. I do see a lot of children with bad reactions to vaccines. We do need them, I do not deny that; but if I can make them safer, I will. And certainly for those who refuse vaccines know Echinacea, not that Echinacea would be a substitute for the vaccines.

Lastly, Echinacea by its nature is an immune enhancer. This should be used in the short term only. Those who suffer from autoimmune disorders must be very cautious using echinacea.

Appendix F

General Wound Care

Wounds vary. Ages, reasons, and results are multiple. Some basics can be applied. Cleanliness is everything, but bleeding and severity must always be kept in mind. See your physician when you have a bad wound. These recommendations are for when you cannot. In those living in remote areas, it wouldn't be a bad idea to get a tetanus shot, they last so long.

With a small basic laceration, allow it to bleed some, enough to cleanse out the wound reasonably. After this, gentle irrigation is important; you do not want to further traumatize damaged tissues. There are times debridement, or the removal of tissue, is important; but that is a topic in itself. Basic abrasions, tears, bruises, injured tissues can be assisted to heal. Irrigate and control bleeding, wrap in sterile gauze or the cleanest wrapping you can find. I keep sterile boxes of gauze for just these occasions. Some wounds require sutures. To prepare a wound to take to a physician, let it bleed some, and rinse gentle, then wrap with the cleanest materials you can find. Control excess bleeding as you can. Small wounds you might be able to treat on your own after thorough cleansing.

Nourish

Naturally, there is a lot you can do. Gently applying olive oil alone to a clean fresh wound is beneficial. Olive oil is very safe and is loaded with unsaturated oils, so essential for cell membranes.

Consider the Exposure

Some wounds are alkaline, and vinegar may be considered before applying nutritive to assist in neutralizing the toxin. Rinse the wound before applying olive oil, or just reapply the olive oil. Insect stings particularly respond to vinegar.

Look, Gently Cleanse, and Treat

For crushed or macerated tissues, after gently cleaning the wound, it is helpful to apply a generous amount of fresh olive oil for its soothing and nourishing properties supports cells very gently. Next I recommend adding a safe herbal such as slippery elm. Slippery elm is loaded with very nutritive elements (chemical constituents) that support flesh regrowth. The late Dr. John Christopher, who any knowledgeable herbalist and naturopath would agree was one of the best, often stated, "Slippery elm becomes flesh." I have seen this in action many times. I am always amazed, and patients are in disbelief and become incredibly hopeful they can learn to manage their health in other ways. I am further amazed at the lack of scar at the end of the course when a wound that is too traumatized to close has the benefit of slippery elm, the inner bark of the somewhat endangered red elm tree. I usually suggest getting slippery elm in capsules as you can be assured there is no mildew risk on a wound. I have purchased quality slippery elm powder in bulk and have kept it frozen years now. I keep some in the refrigerator as well to preserve the bark. It should smell pretty fresh.

If the wound is clean and not bleeding heavily, slippery elm powder dusted generously over the involved area is priceless to healing. Not only that, but the pain is relieved to a remarkable degree as the "new flesh" covers the defect.

These macerated or raw wounds heal well by daily gentle cleansing, application of olive oil or another nonirritant oil followed by the application of slippery elm or other similar type of tissue growth support. Some plants and substitutes are heavy irritants, and this must be watched for.

Dress

The wound should be gentle wrapped in sterile dressing; and if necessary the area should be protected, somewhat immobilized and elevated whenever possible and depending on the severity. With enough slippery elm, the wound will not stick to the dressing. Otherwise it is necessary to use non stick sterile pads under the gauze. There are times that I add a prescription antibiotic to the wound before applying the slippery elm. I use over the counter antibiotics other than neomycin, unless I only have neomycin. I have seen too many contact reactions from neomycin, and this is well documented. This potentially confuses the picture as well slows healing. Often mupirocin ointment is my choice, a prescription topical ointment especially helpful for staph infections so commonly encountered. Finally, Saran Wrap can be useful to occlude wounds and support entry of the nutrients, this should be loosely placed.

Other Considerations

Aloe vera obviously is tremendously therapeutic as well. For burns, especially, aloe stands above all the other plants. Grow your own if you can; the plant does pretty well with little care. The leaves can be frozen if necessary to preserve them. They are cooling, comforting, and cell-structure renewing.

Plantain and mullen both aid in wound healing and could be useful substitutes. Even onion has quercetin, which is very healing to tissues. It depends on what is available. These can be applied in powder or poultice form. Cayenne orally helps control bleeding as well as support circulation to the area. Vitamin E oil topically *after* the wound has healed helps any residual scarring.

APPENDIX G

Mood

To understand mood struggles, you have to remember the story of Bambi, especially when he meets Faline. Rose-colored glasses don't you think? Bambi is walking on air, according to the wise owl. In any event, the euphoria of new love is what I am referring to.

When your friend falls in love, they go on and on about whom they are so drawn to, it is almost irritating some times. They may be well matched but you cannot logic them out of rose-colored glasses any more than they can logic themselves out of rose-colored glasses.

Back to Bambi and Faline; they get married, and they are a good match. But say, he forgets to put the toilet seat down, excuse the metaphor. They are committed for better and for worse, they love each other, but the lenses are now clear.

Depression is gray, or even black, lenses. You cannot logic your way out of it and no one else can either. Counseling helps cope, but it is much handicapped in the face of depression. My goal with antidepressants is to clear the lens. No rose-colored glasses, no automatic bliss here. But antidepressants can help make counseling more effective. You now can see the issues and what you need to do more clearly.

With antidepressants, I believe less is more in many cases. There are so many causes. I have been trying to help alleviate the suffering in alternative ways, and light therapy has helped either as solo therapy or as an adjunct to medications. Although some may benefit from St. John's wort, I am not so impressed with St. John's wort on its' own for depression. St. John's wort may thin blood as well. Many times, depression is just a reaction to a really tough world. Broad spectrum, full day spectrum bulbs and lights are very helpful. I even find blue nanometer light might help with insomnia. Home depot carries these bulbs. Our cool white bulbs kill plants; they are not helpful in maintaining our circadian rhythms. Medications are often needed as the person has so many adaptations and the chemistry is off balance. Cleansing and nutritional approaches in a loving healthful environment contribute to mood. For many, help in the form of pharmaceuticals is necessary. Hopefully, as time goes on and better changes develop, we will be able to find our own happiness and glory to God. We must slow down and pick our priorities. We might need the help of others.

I hope this helps; you would not believe how many times a day I tell the Bambi/Faline version. Think of it more simply as waking up on the right side of the bed.

Appendix H

Easy Digestible Foods

Cooked vegetables are nourishing, alkalinizing, and do not deplete the digestive tract as we process them. Green beans and peas support the adrenals that are often depleted in exhaustion. Onions are especially nutritious and are sources of quercetin necessary for histamine control. Carrots are loaded with nutrition. Beets are blood building. All produce should be washed thoroughly.

Potatoes are nutritious sources of carbohydrates. Although all carbs are now somewhat viewed as bad, it depends on the source. Potatoes are very easy for most to digest and thus to get strength from.

Almond milk and soy milk are preferred over cow's milk. There are too many concerns over cow's milk for me to ignore. Over half of us are deficient in lactase, the enzyme necessary to digest lactose from milk. Yogurt is an exception because of the beneficial bacteria provided, and the fact that yogurt is partially digested. This makes yogurt easier for us to process for the most part.

Berries have so many antioxidant properties that, when possible, they should be included in our daily meals.

Any cool foods might benefit us more if they are chewed and warmed in our mouth prior to swallow. Cooling foods can be depleting. Raw foods should be chewed thoroughly to encourage salivary enzymes to support digestion.

Carrot juice, added with beets or celery juice or maybe some parsley, are very supportive in healing the digestive tract.

Grains to consider include cooked oats and brown rice.

A small amount of red meat, contrary to popular opinion, may help to build someone after they have started plenty of good nutrition. Of course, chicken and fish are good protein sources as well as eggs. We do not need as much protein as we think though. With well-balanced proteins, we only require a couple ounces a day to support ourselves. Nuts have good proteins, but often, people with weak digestions limits their value. Nuts and seeds become irritating to the digestive tract. Nut butters are a good alternative.

We require essential omega acid support to help balance the inflammatory pathways. Omega fatty acids should be stored in a cool place or they can go rancid and smell foul. Good sources of omega oils include supplements of flaxseed (plant source), krill, and salmon. Vitamin D3 is well absorbed when taken with polyunsaturated omega fatty acids such as these. Evening primrose and borage oil also have good nutritional balancing support for the inflammatory pathways. These oils have somewhat different ratios of omega fatty acids.

Herbal teas that help include red raspberry leaf tea (astringent, iron, vitamin C), peppermint (anti-nausea), hyssop (gentle cleansing), hibiscus, and others.

Avoid white products for the most part. The processing in foods is costing us our health. Minimize foods such as breads, pizza, sodas, and in general all artificial substances we call foods. Stevia, a sweet tasting leaf, is a good alternative to sugar. Raw sugar is so much better than brown or white sugar as it provides minerals necessary to process sugar. Blackstrap molasses, available in health food store baking sections, contains plant-based minerals from sugar and can be used to help build up vitality. Gerson recommended a tablespoon three times a week to help build up the health of his cancer patients. He believed in feeding the body not the tumor, so I have followed his recommendations. Blackstrap molasses does have significant potassium, so those with kidney failure must be cautious.

If nausea and pain start, simplify your diet. You may be down to just teas sweetened with honey or raw sugar, even sugar if you need to, for energy until the crisis lets up. Do not become dehydrated as this will slow the resolution of the angry bowel. If the obstruction is more advanced, you will need to be admitted, possibly have surgery, and treated with strong medications that have side effects. Do your best to minimize your risks by being observant. Bowels should move every day. Also realize it is a process to getting the bowel to improve its function; and generally, the longer you have had trouble, the longer it takes to recover. Learn what works for you as an individual.

Trust your intuition and also realize you can improve your vitality.

Elena Suzanne Shea, M.D., M.H.

Education

Texas A&M University, B.S. Biomedical Science, 1983-1987

Texas Tech School of Medicine, M.D. 1988-1992 (top half); research in bipolar, schizophrenia disorder

Baylor Hospital in Dallas, 1992-1993 Internship in Transitional Anesthesia (rotating internship), research in alopecia post-operatively

The School of Natural Healing in Provo, Utah, Master Herbalist, June, 2002

Southwest Oklahoma Family Practice Residency, July 2006 to June, 2009.

2010 ABFM

Index

CPSIA information can be obtained at www.ICGtesting.com
Printed in the USA
LVOW12s2105080914

403050LV00001B/143/P